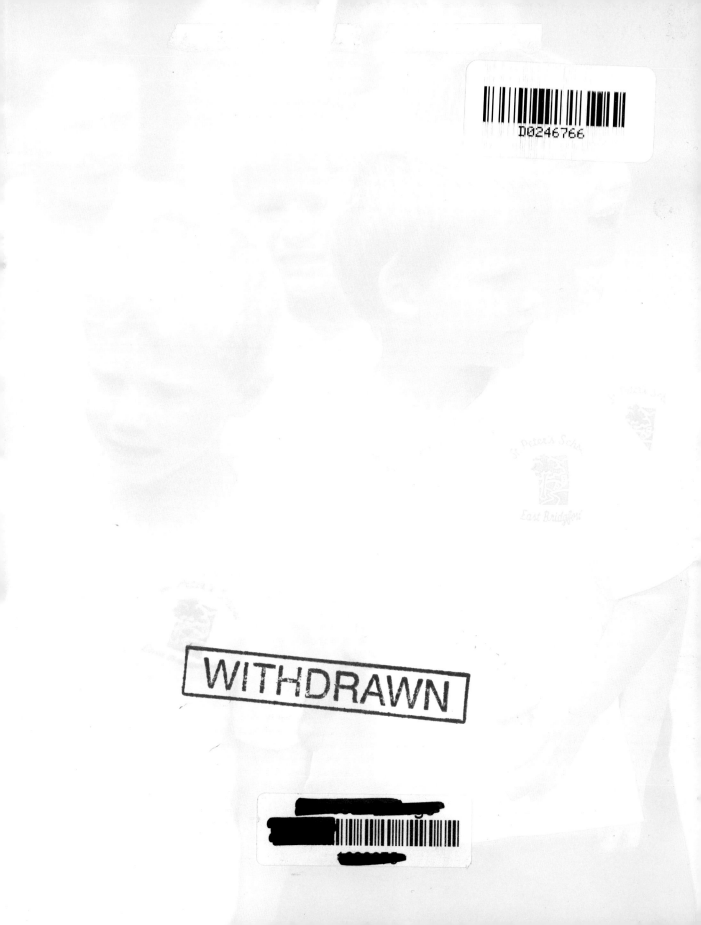

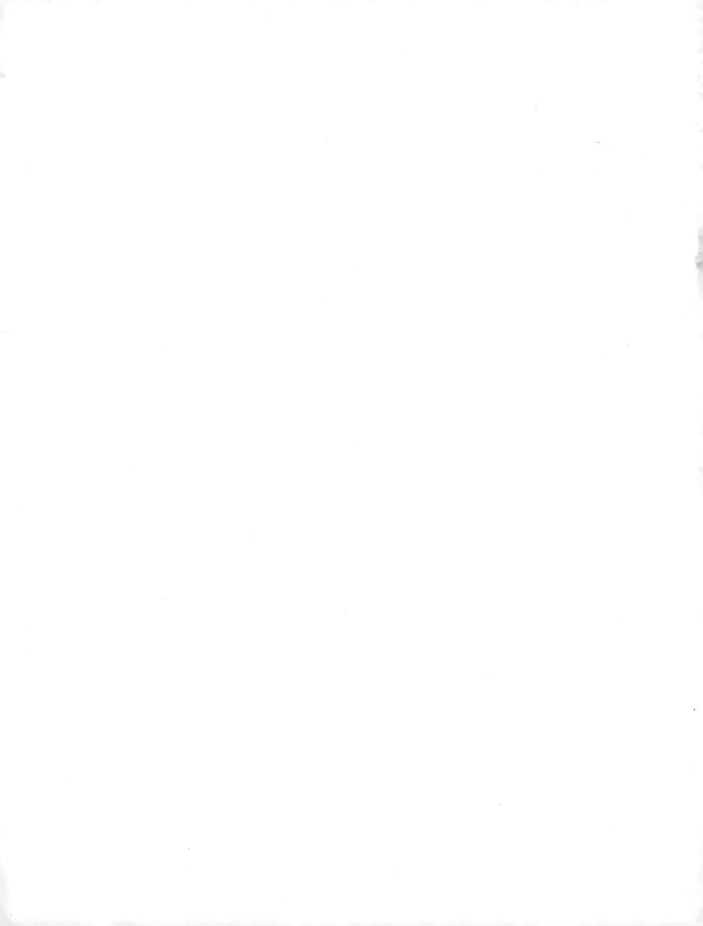

THE DINNER LADY

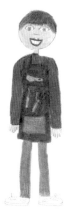

'She's an inspiration to us all – the more people who listen to her, the better the chances are of our children eating well.'

Hugh Fearnley-Whittingstall

'Jeanette Orrey – about to become a legend in your children's lunchtime.'

Fat Nation, BBC1

'This book is packed full of tasty, healthy and simple recipes using the best possible ingredients. Your children will thank you for buying it.'

Antony Worrall Thompson

'Jeanette Orrey is a dynamo, a true pioneer … Every school cook and parent interested in food needs this book.'

Felicity Lawrence, author of
Not On the Label: What really goes into the food on your plate

'Jeanette's unique and unchallengeable authority is that she is a dinner lady – and what she knows from her own experience has commanded respect at the highest level and triggered a food revolution. She is living proof that one person who has a combination of energy and the right ideas at the right time can quite literally change the world. Jeanette Orrey is an inspiration.'

Patrick Holden, director of the Soil Association

'A fantastic, stimulating book, from an inspirational woman who has proved that the impossible can be achieved – decent food, healthy kids and a school meals budget that works. A revolution in the quality of school meals is long overdue. Jeanette is in the vanguard of that revolution, showing us all how it can be done! They say that big changes only happen as a result of the action of dedicated individuals. Jeanette is going to change the way our children eat.'

Lizzie Vann, founder of Organix Brands plc

'I wish school dinners in my day had tasted as good as the meals dished up by Jeanette and her team. I have had lunch at St Peter's and know what nutritious, varied meals the pupils are enjoying. By using locally produced meat, fruit and veg, Jeanette is giving local farmers and growers a fair crack of the whip.'

Lord Larry Whitty, Department for Environment, Food and Rural Affairs (Defra)

'Jeanette is a lady who believes strongly in what she is doing and is not prepared to take no for an answer easily. She has proved that it is possible to serve high-quality, locally sourced British food and has re-established the school lunch as a meal to look forward to.'

Sir Ben Gill, former president of the NFU

'Most movements for change start with a new idea, with a theory about how to make the world a better place. Jeanette started the movement to make school meals fun, tasty and healthy by doing it. As a result, thousands of children are now eating healthier, fresher, tastier food for their school dinner. Nothing is as likely to change what people do faster than seeing a better system actually working. That is why what Jeanette has achieved at St Peter's has been so influential. We have a long way to go before all children are served the unprocessed, locally sourced and where available organic food that they have a right to expect, and that they need for healthy development. With Jeanette to inspire us, we will get there.'

Lord Peter Melchett, Soil Association

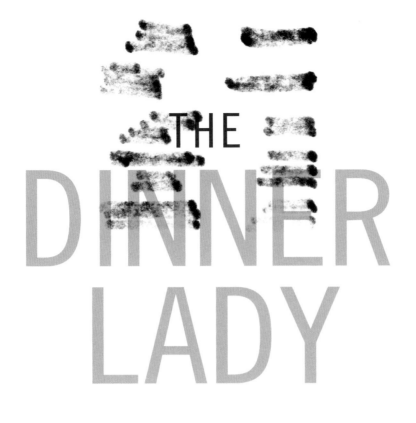

THE
DINNER
LADY

JEANETTE ORREY

WITH SUSAN FLEMING

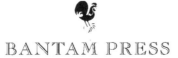

BANTAM PRESS

LONDON · TORONTO · SYDNEY · AUCKLAND · JOHANNESBURG

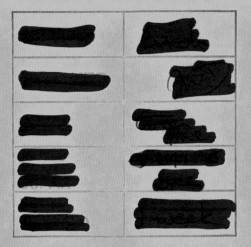

TRANSWORLD PUBLISHERS
61–63 Uxbridge Road, London W5 5SA
a division of The Random House Group Ltd

RANDOM HOUSE AUSTRALIA (PTY) LTD
20 Alfred Street, Milsons Point, Sydney,
New South Wales 2061, Australia

RANDOM HOUSE NEW ZEALAND LTD
18 Poland Road, Glenfield, Auckland 10, New Zealand

RANDOM HOUSE SOUTH AFRICA (PTY) LTD
Endulini, 5a Jubilee Road, Parktown 2193, South Africa

Published 2005 by Bantam Press
a division of Transworld Publishers

Copyright © Jeanette Orrey 2005
Design: Fiona Andreanelli; Nicky Barneby
Food Stylist: Sue Ashworth
Home Economist: Caroline Marson

A catalogue record for this book is available
from the British Library.
ISBN 0593 054296

Printed by Butler & Tanner, Frome, Somerset

3 5 7 9 10 8 6 4 2

Papers used by Transworld Publishers are natural, recyclable products
made from wood grown in sustainable forests. The manufacturing processes conform
to the environmental regulations of the country of origin.

1080675
£16.99

Contents

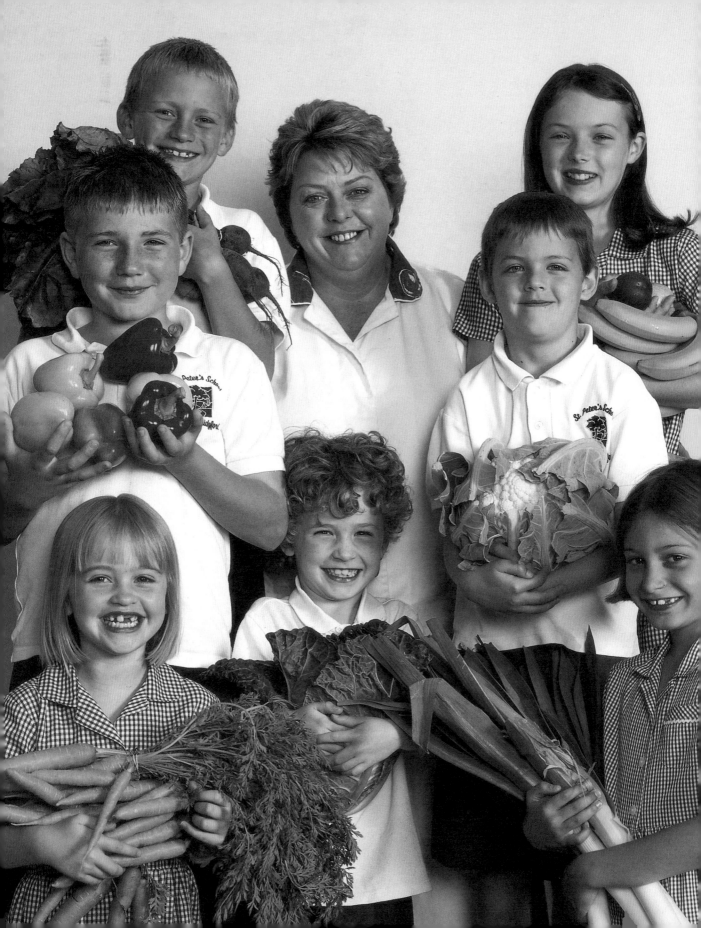

To my three sons, Gareth, William
and Jonathan, with all my love

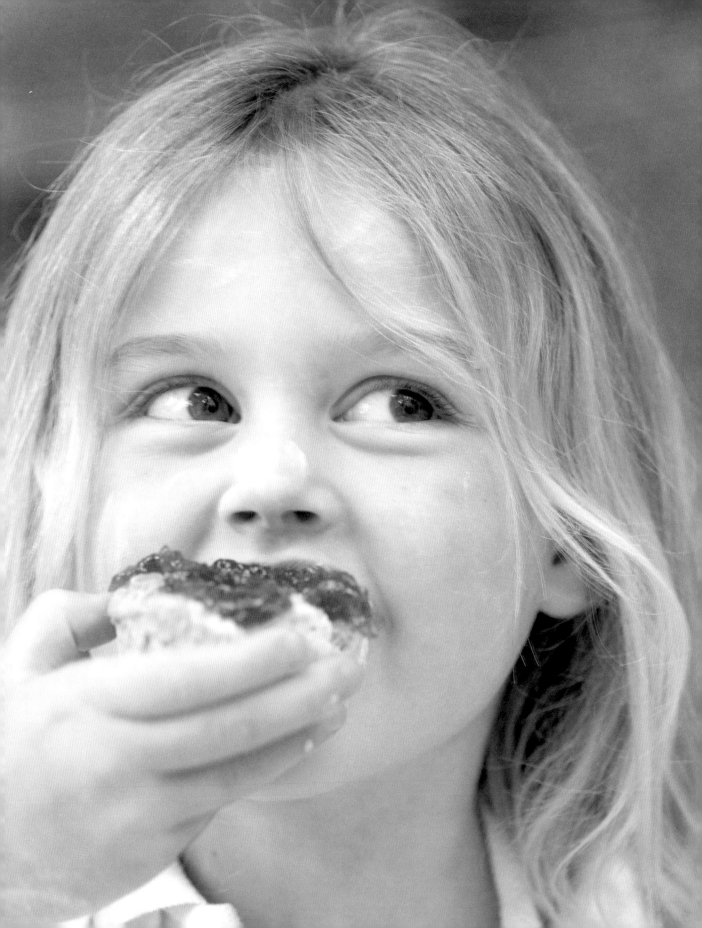

Hallelujah – finally a book from a dinner lady!

For the last year and a half I've been working on a project about school dinners, learning about all the deep and mysterious things that go into the feeding of our nation of kids. Very early on, me and my team became aware of the amazing work of Jeanette Orrey at St Peter's School in Nottinghamshire. I suppose you would call her a local hero, and now that she's been seconded by the Soil Association (the people who help farmers achieve and maintain organic status in their food production – i.e., normal food without any horrible chemicals) she's become a national hero, going round schools and showing dinner ladies the way.

If you're a parent buying this book, you might think that changing school dinners would be simple, but oh no – you couldn't be more wrong! On my own school dinners journey I've seen exactly what Jeanette must have had to overcome, which is getting the head teacher, all the other teaching staff, the parents, the kids, the council and the suppliers onside. Not an easy job. It involves patience and creativity, and when coming up against authorities whose current systems Jeanette's clearly outshining, you need to be really brave and confident as well, and, quite frankly, only care about the kids.

What I also found impressive about Jeanette is that she now spends a lot of her time teaching other schools about how they can change their bloomin' awful rubbish food into hearty food that's going to make the kids healthier and brighter. You probably don't realize how important the example of her kitchen is. Nutritionally these are really dark times in Britain – we're the laughing stock of Europe, healthwise. We need more people like Jeanette – and her headmaster at St Peter's, David Maddison – who are feeding the kids up in those so-important early years so that their bones, immune systems and bodies really do have a better chance. And not only has Jeanette written this book for other dinner ladies, but for home use too. She gives clever, constructive recipes (which give quantities for 4 or 96!) so that parents will be able to make simple, nutritious meals for their children.

This year I've experienced some truly amazing transformations of children and families, all through food, and yet people still find it difficult to understand that what you put in your mouth can change you so much.

Well done, babe. This book is another step to showing people the way.

Jamie Oliver

Foreword

Introduction

WHEN I SET OUT on my journey as a school dinner lady, I never thought I would end up trying to actually change the way that children eat – but then, admittedly, I have always been someone who speaks her own mind and gets things done. And, something much more to the point, I have always been passionate about good, honest British food – fresh meat and fish, seasonal fresh fruit and vegetables. This was what I fed my own family – my husband and three strapping boys (all now over six feet) – and it's what I think all children should be eating.

Since those days, though – and my eldest son is now in his mid-twenties – the concept of family eating seems to have been eroded. As a child I accepted without question what my mother and grandmother put in front of me at mealtimes, and we all ate together daily at the kitchen table. I expected nothing less of my own children when they arrived. Today, families are more fragmented. Parents feel they have no time to cook, so resort to ready meals (which, of course, weren't around twenty-five years ago). Children have been introduced in the meantime to foods specially 'created' for them (those weren't around either), and many eat these – away from the sociability of the kitchen table – in front of the television. I may have started a mini revolution in schools, but if I could do the same in people's homes for family meals – reintroducing the principles of good food, good eating, good fellowship and tasty, practical recipes – I would be a very happy woman.

When I first started working in schools, the food was basically good, if a little boring. But over the years, bureaucracy – and economics – took over, and the food we were allowed to serve in school began to suffer. What government deemed 'best value' unfortunately meant the cheapest, and packet mixes, pre-cut and pre-packed vegetables and frozen 'free-flow' meat (probably from several different animals, and even more countries) became the norm. Thus began the era of the processed dinner. We dinner ladies became demoralized and de-skilled – you don't need much in the way of a brain to scissor open a packet, do you? – and many children, for whom that school dinner might be the only substantial meal of the day, were not, to my mind, being fed properly. I was at my wits' end trying to find ways of serving what I call *real* food, not highly processed food.

My chance finally came in April 2000. The government of the day had passed national legislation the year before which allowed secondary schools three options for running their catering services. They could either continue to use the local authority system (which is what we had been doing), get an external company to provide the whole service for them, or they could run every aspect of the process themselves. When the choice was extended to primary schools, with the help and support of the headmaster, the school governors and my ladies in the kitchen, we decided to 'go it alone'. And, five years later, we have succeeded in more ways than I could have thought possible.

My original intention was simply to provide good fresh food for my school dinners. I didn't dream that that quest would involve me in contributing substantially to the local economy (by sourcing local produce), and becoming closely involved with the organic movement (I now work part-time for the Soil Association). I didn't dream that I would or could become so involved with the children, the parents and the school itself – I am 'only a dinner lady' after all – but my ideas and passions have filtered into many of the school classes, and food has become an integral part of the curriculum. I have seen those children 'grow' in knowledge, and because they (and their families) are now so aware of the principles of good food and eating, I think they are well on the way to becoming healthy adults, avoiding common nutritional ills such as obesity, high blood pressure, diabetes, and even some types of cancer.

And that is what I hope this book will teach you and your children at home. We all want to give our children the best start in life, and obviously food plays a key role in their development, both of body and of brain. Children, more than any other age group, 'are what they eat'. With today's increasing time pressures for parents and children alike, preparing a good, home-cooked meal might seem daunting, especially when there are so many ready meals available. But cooking at home is so satisfying, and can be so much fun. Involving the children, too, is important – they're never too young to help or to learn – and by eating together as a family, you are laying the foundation for a lifetime of health, pleasure and sociability. They may have their likes and dislikes, and fussy ways, but don't despair. Children will eat when, what and how much they like (often less, to be honest, than you think they might need), but yours is still the most valuable input. I know what I am talking about, because I was a mother before I was a school dinner lady – and there are a few pointers in these pages that might help you.

My story is nothing special so far as I am concerned, and the message I have been 'preaching' is certainly not rocket science. It's just common sense. Good, nutritious food is easy to obtain (once you know how) and easy to cook (I promise). The recipes here may be plain, but they are tasty, and not at all difficult to make in the home kitchen. Most importantly though, they have all been tried and tested – and approved – by that most notoriously difficult group of all – the children themselves.

Jeanette Orrey

PART 1

Just a
Dinner Lady

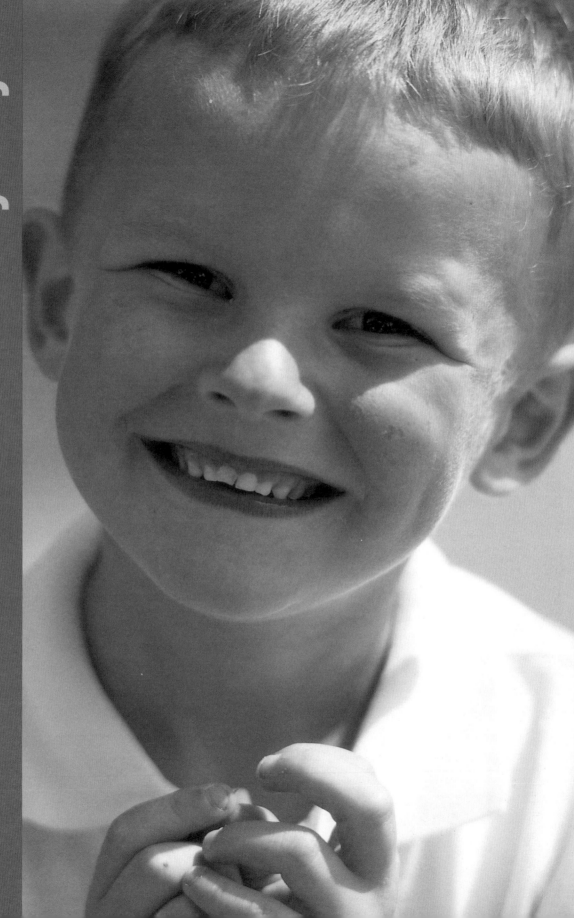

MY LOVE OF FOOD began when I was very young – as it should for every child. I grew up in the countryside in Nottinghamshire, and was surrounded by family, Mum and Dad, later my brother Robert, and two sets of grandparents. We were all very close, and I feel very fortunate still that I have so many family members living not too far away. I think it's a rarity nowadays.

When Mum and Dad weren't working – they ran a milk round at first, then the post office in Elston (where I still live) – we would spend time together. We would go for drives in the car, we would go shopping for food and clothes in local markets, and we visited and had tea with both sets of grandparents. We also all used to eat together as a family. There was the occasional row, of course, and something that I *didn't* want to eat, but I have always felt that my passion for good food today – and my ability to put that passion across – stems from those meals and conversations around our kitchen table at home.

I used to love going to Grandma's particularly, because everything tasted so good. She always cooked traditional staples like meat and gravy, boiled potatoes and vegetables followed by something like rice pudding with a blob of jam, which I thought was fantastic, even on the days when her rice was lumpy! Part of the reason that her dinners were so good was that most of the ingredients were home grown, so I got used to the best from a very early age. Grandad had two allotments where he grew vegetables, as well as a garden where he kept chickens for fresh eggs, and a cockerel to fatten up for Christmas lunch every year (my Dad to this day prefers cockerel to turkey at Christmas). Grandma never needed to buy potatoes or vegetables, as they were always dug fresh from the ground (there is *such* a difference in flavour; if only all of us could grow our own). Once I started at school, I used to go to Grandma's rather than stay for school dinner. I remember looking forward to it – I was usually so hungry after a morning of concentrating (well, trying to). That always kept me going through the afternoon, until the end of the school day. On my way home I loved to pop into Archer's when I could. It was a proper old-fashioned sweet shop in the village with huge glass jars filled with multi-coloured boiled sweets. And then, when I got home, Mum would probably have a home-made cake or some scones to have with a cup of tea.

Starting to Cook

MUM COOKED IN MUCH the same way as Grandma, never very adventurous, but tasty and fresh, good traditional English cooking. I helped her in the kitchen whenever I could, but I never considered cooking as a life or career option. I used to peel, stir and mix; and we made pastry, scones and what we called 'cut-and-come-again cakes', fruit cakes that seemed to last for ever. Apparently Mum would go 'tut' as I'd mix the sugar, marge, egg and flour for a Victoria sponge, then eat half of the sweet, gooey mixture before it ever saw the tin! We all used to cook cakes and biscuits much more then than we do now, all over the country, and home-made stuff always tastes so much better than bought. I think it's a pity that we've lost sight of what is actually a long-standing British tradition, and we also seem to have lost one of the nicest meals, high tea.

Later, I was taught how to cook at school, but I absolutely hated it. Well, I didn't much like school anyway. I wasn't ever very academic, and my reports always used to say, 'Could do better' and 'Has got it, but doesn't use it' … I can remember the cookery teacher even now, a Miss Dixon.

… the first meal I cooked for George was fish fingers, chips and peas.

She was very old-fashioned, and very critical, and she used to tell me that I would never be able to make pastry. Once, in sheer temper, I threw the brown leaden lump that I had been working on across the room, and it landed right in the middle of the bun on the top of her head. I was a trainee Gordon Ramsay even then … Now, however, I love making pastry: it's very relaxing, even in a frantic school kitchen.

The first time I had to cook for someone else was when I got married, at the age of eighteen. I'd met George at the local youth club in Elston a couple of years before, just after I'd left school. I was serving an apprenticeship as a hairdresser, and he, a year older than me, was an apprentice stonemason, helping to renovate Southwell Minster. I'd done bits and bobs of cooking at home, of course, but I had never actually made a complete meal. I'm ashamed to say that the first meal I cooked for George was fish fingers, chips and peas. He looked at me, and then he looked at his dinner and said, 'What's this?' I should have known better as his mother, Evelyn, like my mother, had always cooked 'good proper food', as George would call it. So I thought, whoops, I think I'd better do something about this.

I pulled my socks up by reading cookery books. I found the Be-Ro flour book very helpful, with recipes for quiches, pies, pastries etc. I thought, right, I'm going to have a good go at this. Thinking about recipes got my imagination going, and what with asking and getting advice on meat cookery from the butcher, and endless tips from my Mum, I must admit that I started to enjoy it. Then I saw an evening course advertised at the local college in Newark. That course, on basic cookery – white sauces, mince, grilling, making stews etc. – was what really started the ball rolling, and then there was no stopping me. After that, I enrolled in a second, more advanced course, which was about dinner-party cooking. That wasn't quite my thing, but I learned a lot; I now know all the basic principles, which I can use if need be. (I also enjoyed getting out in the evenings, and the company of the other girls – because they were all girls, of course.) I was so keen that two years later I went back to enrol again, to find that, to my disappointment, the Home Economics department had been scrapped and replaced with Information Technology.

But it didn't stop me cooking. I'm still a fairly plain cook, although I love experimenting – but it's all English. If I have a basic stew, I'll put something extra in it, but never anything outrageous – perhaps a little curry powder occasionally, but there's not a lemongrass stalk in sight! A friend of mine has a saying, 'Chop it up and chuck it in', and that happily sums up how many of us tend to cook at home. It was especially relevant for me as I soon had to cook for a family, for George and I went on to have three sons in the first ten years or so of our marriage, Gareth, William and Jonathan.

Good Food from the Start

I HAVE BEEN FEEDING CHILDREN – three of my own, and hundreds of other people's – for over twenty-five years now. Children are contrary creatures so far as food is concerned, and mothers, who want to do the best for their offspring, can become desperate if a baby spits out his carrots, if a toddler won't eat lumpy food, or an older child won't eat vegetables. Whereas Tony Blair said, 'Education, education, education', I say, 'Perseverance, perseverance, perseverance'.

Starting solid food

When you are weaning babies off milk alone, the fun can begin. There are lots of baby foods you can buy in jars and packets, and some are very good indeed, particularly organic varieties. Interestingly, half of all baby food sold these days is organic, and it is thought that three out of four children eat some organic food during their first year. Why? Is it just a fad, or do parents really trust in foods that are labelled organic, believing that the foods do not contain certain harmful substances? I believe it's the latter. However, I had my boys at a time when the choice was more limited than it is now. So I just cooked for them myself, the simplest possible purées at first, then tiny portions of family food later. (Well, this was the intention, but I must admit that Gareth was such a hungry baby that I was feeding him Weetabix and milk at about six to eight weeks. The health visitor was appalled…) Cooking foods yourself is much more economical, especially at the beginning, as they will be taking only a teaspoon or so – and the rest of a jar of baby food might be wasted.

There are many books that can advise on weaning much better than this one, but there are a few basic tips I can remember. Because I am used to boys, I have used 'him' and 'he' when talking about babies/children, but of course it equally applies to 'her' and 'she'.

🍽 Don't start offering solid food until babies are about six months, or they have at least doubled their birth weight – when they require more energy and nutrients than milk alone can supply. If solid food is offered too early, a baby's digestive system might not be ready to deal with a new food, and the baby could develop a food intolerance or allergy (see the box on pages 62–3).

🍽 The texture has to be right – a purée could have some breast or formula milk or boiled water added to make it soft and wet. (Anything too sticky might frighten a baby.) Strain out any skin or seeds, which the baby cannot digest.

🍽 Try soft cooked puréed vegetables and fruit first (see the box on page 20).

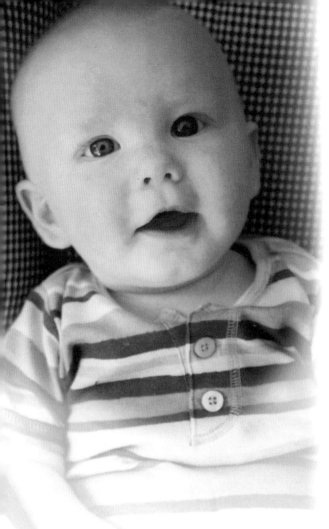

could be half asleep by this stage, give him a quarter of his milk, or enough to remove the initial pangs of hunger. Always remember that you know your own baby best, and each baby is different.

🍽 Try only a teaspoon at first, and try only one food at a time to make sure it suits your baby. Be prepared for him to make a few funny faces or spit it out, for both texture and taste are completely unfamiliar.

🍽 When you make a purée for the baby, you don't have to do so in tiny amounts. Make more than you need at one meal, and freeze the rest in ice-cube trays – a good baby portion size. But remember to defrost it in time!

🍽 Once solid foods are more established, you can offer the baby a food to eat in his hand – a piece of cooked carrot, for instance, or a chunk of raw peeled apple. Things to chew on, even without teeth, are good, because they help the gums and jaw (see pages 84–5). Never leave a baby alone with a finger food, though, as he could easily 'bite' off more than he can chew, and choke.

🍽 Do not add salt or sugar to any food.

🍽 Baby rice cereal or puréed home-cooked rice is the best to offer at first because of potential allergy problems with other grains.

🍽 Give him at least half of his milk before you try to feed him a little solid food. His hunger will be satisfied, and he might therefore be more sociable and actually interested in trying something different. Or if you have a dozy baby, who

🍽 One of the world's largest and longest-running medical studies ('Children of the 90s', officially known as the Avon Longitudinal Study of Parents and Children, or ALSPAC), has come up with many fascinating findings in its first fourteen years: one is that babies who are not introduced to solid food until after the age of nine months are more likely to turn into fussy eaters.

If you have patience at this very early stage, you will be rewarded in heaven – or at least in the future, because you will have a child who relishes new flavours, who enjoys good food, and who enjoys eating.

FIRST BABY FOODS

SIX TO SEVEN MONTHS (all foods cooked, and finely puréed)

Cereals	Baby rice only at first (available in packets).
Vegetables	Carrots first, later other roots such as parsnips, swede, turnip, celeriac. Green vegetables such as courgettes, beans, celery, fennel, peas, broccoli. Fruit vegetables such as tomatoes.
Fruits	Cooked apples and pears first, then apricots, cherries, peaches, nectarines, plums, kiwi, mango, papaya. Raw apple could be tried, and reconstituted and cooked dried fruit. Acidic fruits such as citrus and pineapples should be avoided in the early weaning stage.
Eggs	Eggs are good protein, but avoid until eight months, especially if allergies run in the family.
White meats	Chicken and turkey without skin.
Red meats	Beef, veal, lamb and offal, without fat.
Dairy foods	Avoid until later, although plain yoghurt can be tolerated.
Fish	Not yet.
Finger foods	Chunks of raw or cooked apple, carrot, fingers of baked bread.

SEVEN TO NINE MONTHS (foods cooked and raw, less finely puréed)

Cereals Cereals other than rice can be tried, but not if allergies run in the family. Pasta, rice and bread.

Vegetables Cooked green vegetables such as cabbage, as well as potatoes, beetroot, some pulses (lentils), sweet potatoes. Watercress and avocado could be eaten raw.

Fruits Citrus fruits, cherries, apricots, peaches, nectarines, melon and pineapple could be raw.

Eggs Try some cooked egg yolk only at eight to nine months, but only if there are no allergies in the family.

Meats As before, but avoid frying, and try to use good-quality meat. Avoid processed meats such as sausages, bacon, pies and pastries, which are high in salt, fat and additives.

Dairy foods Hard cheeses can be enjoyed, but avoid cooking them (the protein toughens). Soft cottage cheeses are good too, but avoid unpasteurized cheeses, because of the fears of listeria. Yoghurt could have fruit added, but avoid bought fruit yoghurts, which can contain a huge amount of sugar.

Fish Steam or bake white fish only, if no allergies in the family. Avoid smoked and oily fish, and all shellfish. Remove skin, and look carefully for bones.

Finger foods Chunks of raw apple, carrot, celery, cucumber, fennel, etc. Fingers of baked bread.

NINE TO FIFTEEN MONTHS (foods cooked and raw, chopped)

Cereals
Unsweetened cereals such as Weetabix and Shredded Wheat could be offered, as well as puffed wheat or porridge. Pasta, rice, bread and perhaps couscous.

Vegetables
As before, but now pulses can be eaten – including baked beans! Sweetcorn, onions, peppers and salads will be enjoyed.

Fruits
Cooked berries, raw strawberries (go easy because of possible reactions), seedless grapes (but only if he can chew well).

Eggs
Whole eggs can be eaten at twelve months. Scrambled, boiled, hard-boiled, omelettes, etc.

Meats
As before, with as little fat as possible. Pork and ham could now be included, as well as game.

Dairy foods
After 12 months, most experts say a child could be moved from breast or formula on to cows' milk. Otherwise, as before.

Fish
White fish only still.

Finger foods
As before, but he will probably be fingering *all* his foods now, as he attempts to feed himself!

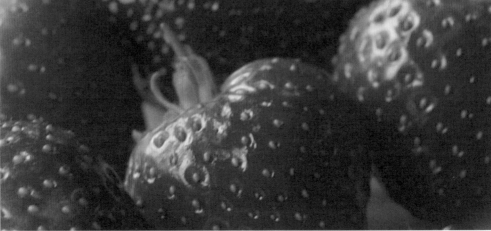

Pre-school children at home

Until he or she goes to school, most of what a child eats will have been chosen by you, so make sure that it is good food. It is adults who choose and buy food, not children. Sadly, however, children are often introduced to biscuits, ice cream and lollies, sweets, chips and crisps during these pre-school years (by friends, grannies, and in restaurants and through television advertising), but try to limit these as much as possible. They are usually not very nutritious, and can very easily become a major part of an under-five's intake, which means that more valuable foods might be ignored or refused.

Again, although it was a long time ago, there are a few things I can remember. I've written them in no particular order, or age group, so some are not particularly relevant to slightly older children. The most important thing as far as I am concerned is to eat together as a family, at least once a day, and to make a habit of this from the very earliest stages. Gareth had a high chair in which he sat with us while George and I had breakfast. He ate earlier than us in the evening, but I still sat with him at the table. When the other two arrived, the high chair was assigned to the youngest, and the older boy(s) sat on proper chairs at the table (fat cushions came in handy). I had been taught that eating and sitting down at table went together, so there was never any question of an alternative (such as sneaking off to watch TV with a plate or tray on one's knee). I'm very much in favour of children eating with grown-ups – they learn many social skills from being with others – and indeed with their brothers and sisters. Children copy other people, especially other children, and if they can see them eating with enjoyment, even potentially fussy eaters will get the message eventually.

◉ Grown-up food, cut up for a very young child, can be higher in fat, salt and sugar than the carefully prepared purées of before, so cook family meals carefully – it will benefit you as well.

◉ Always put very much less on a child's plate – and use a smaller plate so that everything is in proportion. We do this at St Peter's with our pre-school and early years. I don't want to 'over-face' a small child with a huge plate. Cooking in small dishes can be appealing – try individual shepherd's pies or fruit crumbles in ramekin dishes.

◉ Don't offer too many snacks between meals. These can fill a child up, making them less interested in eating proper food at the proper time. Sweet foods, like biscuits, will give them energy and fill a 'hole', but the blood-sugar level drops too quickly, resulting in tiredness and bad temper. This is particularly true of toddlers, who are notoriously demanding and notoriously grumpy. A piece of apple or carrot would be much better than a biscuit.

◉ Don't worry about 'table manners' too early. If a toddler feels happier eating with his fingers, let him. But he must be able to manage a knife, fork and spoon properly by the time he goes to school. I've seen far too many children who don't know how, and not only does it make work for the midday supervisors, who look after the children during the lunch break, it's rather humiliating for the child himself.

◉ I found with my boys that one of the worst things to do was make comments about the food I was just about to serve them. 'This will make you strong' or 'It's good for you' made them much more resistant to eating it, for some reason. My mother's favourite saying with my youngest son, Jonathan, was 'Eat your crusts, it'll make your hair curl'. He is now eighteen, and won't eat crusts, as he still doesn't want curly hair…

◉ Serve fruit after a meal, or give just a small quantity of a pudding or dessert. Never bribe a reluctant meat or veg eater with the promise of pudding or a sweet thing to come if he eats everything up. This will reinforce the idea that sweet things are more desirable.

◉ Putting foods in dishes on the table, for people to help themselves from, is often better for children, even the smallest. They can choose what and how much they want to eat, and they can always come back for more. Even at school age, I see lots of children eating more salad than they might have intended, because everything is there for them to choose from by themselves.

◉ By serving home-cooked foods from the start, that is what children will think of as 'proper' food, and hopefully they will react adversely to commercial foods with their concentrated saltiness or sweetness.

◉ Don't make food a big issue, because so many more children, at a much younger age, are suffering from eating disorders.

◉ If food is refused or just picked at for a long time, don't force the issue. A child will eat when he is hungry, and can't be forced to eat. Mealtimes should never be a battleground, and good food is about *enjoying*.

Reluctant vegetable eaters

Many parents worry that their children don't like or eat vegetables, especially green vegetables, which are an important part of the diet. A number of vegetables have a strong, slightly bitter flavour, so it is not totally surprising, given that sweet tastes are generally preferred. Often the flavour of a vegetable becomes stronger through overcooking – something we British are, sadly, rather internationally known for – so careful cooking could be the answer. Hopefully, though, if you have given a baby fresh, well-cooked vegetables from the start, the problem won't arise.

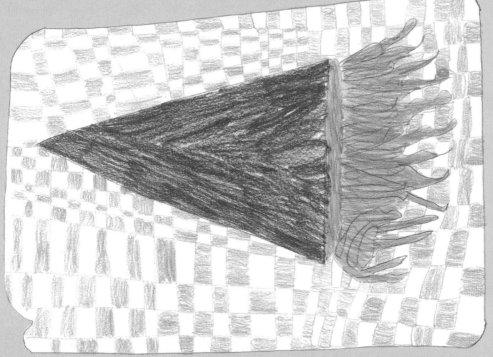

◉ If anyone else in the family doesn't like a particular vegetable, try to 'retrain' them before the baby or under five-year-old can copy.

◉ Try to offer a *selection* of carefully cooked vegetables, so that everyone can choose something that is liked, and try to vary the cooking method from day to day.

◉ Cook green vegetables until just tender. Some vegetables can be steamed rather than boiled, which can improve flavour and appearance: broccoli and carrot, for instance. Cut them up into small pieces or slices – Brussels sprouts, for instance, will be much less challenging if sliced.

◉ Stir-frying is good for vegetables, and they are always less soggy than if boiled. You can cook a selection of colourful vegetables together with some flavouring, such as soy sauce.

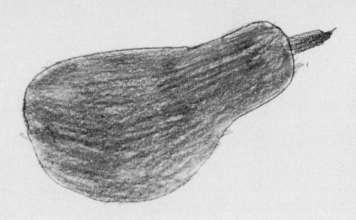

Roasted vegetables are always popular. Pumpkin or squash is good, responding much better – and much more tastily – to this process than to boiling or steaming. Try roasting parsnips with the Sunday joint; their caramelized sweetness will be much appreciated. Roast tomatoes, especially cherry tomatoes, are very popular at St Peter's (see page 193).

Vegetable purées are appealing – something you can do with all root vegetables (potatoes, parsnips, carrots, celeriac, swede, beetroot, turnip), and with pumpkin, cauliflower, broccoli, Brussels sprouts. You could mix purées too, which can result in some amazing and appealing colour combinations.

If you grow your own veg, or have fresh supplies near by, freeze what you can't use if you have a glut. Freeze them raw or blanched, and you should follow the instructions in a good freezing book. You can serve them as an out-of-season treat.

Take the puréed veg idea one step further, and serve it as a soup, which can be topped with chopped herbs, or tiny bread croûtons baked in the oven for texture. Or make the soup more chunky, perhaps adding some soup-sized pasta.

Make food look colourful and attractive on the plate, by using a variety of different coloured foods. Think of the effect of, say, tiny sprigs of broccoli and cauliflower with chunks of red or yellow peppers in a stir-fry.

Children like finger foods – dunking soldiers in boiled eggs, for instance – so try offering small pots of nutritious dips with fingers of vegetables or fruit such as carrot, celery, cucumber or apple. They might like dipping asparagus stalks into melted butter, or the 'poor man's alternative', sprouting broccoli.

'Disguising' food is a good way of getting a reluctant small or large eater to try different things. Two of my sons don't like mushrooms, but they don't recognize them when they are cooked and puréed in a vegetable soup. Mashed potato could be mixed with other cooked mashed vegetables for a change – try swede, turnips, celeriac or parsnip. Many vegetables can be puréed into a sauce for pasta, or into a gravy (where they won't be noticed), as I do at St Peter's. A lot of the children don't care for onions, so I cook them, purée them and put them into the gravy for a roast.

'Hide' vegetables in a stew, lasagne or pasta sauce, or in a potato-cake-like dish to be fried or baked, such as bubble and squeak.

Stuff vegetables with a tasty or attractive filling and bake them: try peppers, tomatoes, courgettes, aubergines. Stuffed tomatoes, or lengths of celery with a 'stuffing', could be served uncooked.

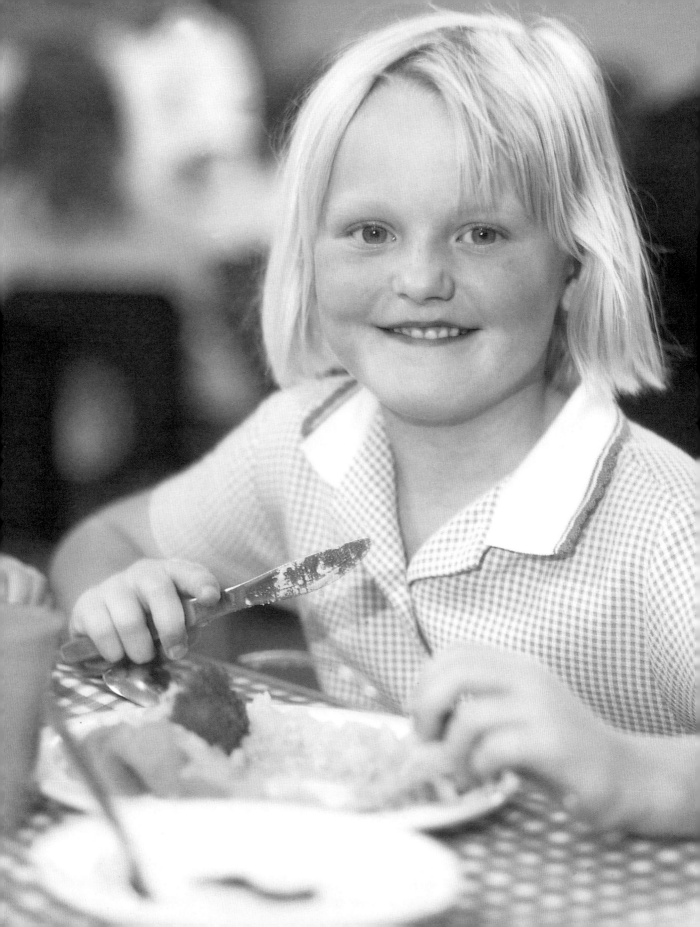

Reluctant fruit eaters

This is usually less of a problem than vegetables. Fruits are generally sweeter than vegetables, thus are more readily accepted – and quite a few fruits are seen as a treat anyway (strawberries, for example).

🍽 Make sure that any fruit you offer is fully ripe. Unripe fruits can be hard, sourer in flavour and can even cause stomach upsets, because they are less digestible.

🍽 Always have a selection of fruit on offer (a better alternative for a snack than a biscuit).

🍽 Fresh fruit at the end of a meal is a good alternative to a pudding – although there are lots of cooked fruit dishes that will be very much appreciated.

🍽 A platter of bite-sized pieces of fruit, single or mixed, can be forked by all the family – watermelon, for instance. Or you can mix fruit in a bowl for a fruit salad (see page 222).

🍽 Take children to pick their own fruit (if you don't grow fruit yourself in the garden). This was always a treat for my boys. PYO farms are all over the place now, in season. Go blackberrying in autumn. Blackberries grow almost everywhere, even in towns (although don't pick too near a road because of the potential lead hazard).

🍽 As with vegetables, mix good colours together in a dish to make it look more appealing. A colourful fruit salad is a prime example, and you could mix some fruit together for breakfast and top with yoghurt.

🍽 Mixing fruit with yoghurt, puréeing it first or leaving it in chunks, is a great way of encouraging fruit eating. Plain yoghurt is a good thing for children to eat anyway – but avoid bought fruit yoghurts, as one tub can contain up to a tablespoon of sugar.

🍽 You can freeze pieces of fruit – bananas, for instance – and they can be eaten as an 'ice lolly'.

🍽 Make softer fruits into a sauce (the posh word is 'coulis') to go over other fruits or some ice cream. Raspberries, blackberries, peaches, apricots and nectarines are good for this.

🍽 Make fruit into a juice. Citrus fruit can be squeezed easily; some others might need to be juiced in a special machine. Add fizzy or still water to dilute if necessary.

🍽 Roasting fruit like pineapple or banana slices, or frying them in a little butter, can make them taste more appetizing.

🍽 Put chunks of fruit on to a skewer to make them look different.

Cooking for Others

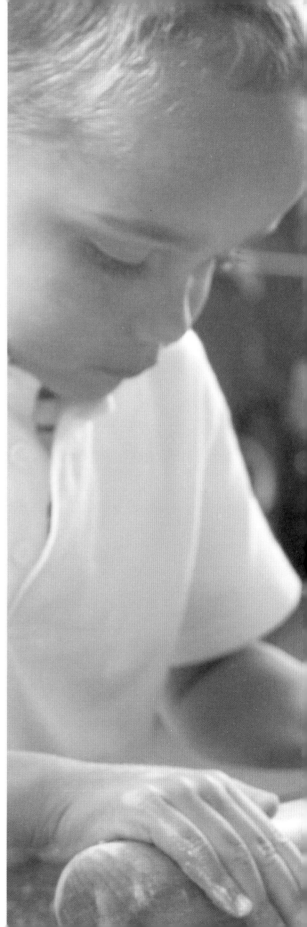

IN 2004, GEORGE AND I celebrated our thirtieth wedding anniversary. George is a quiet, unassuming man, who works very hard. When he was made redundant from stone-masonry, he decided to go down the mines, and he has been there ever since, working in one of the few remaining collieries in Nottinghamshire. Our life together has had its ups and downs, but we're still a strong unit – and he manages to rein me in ever so occasionally! Having four men in the household, I soon had to learn how to put tasty, satisfying meals on the table. I used to do all my shopping at the local butcher, greengrocer and village shop – we all did in those days – and made everything from scratch, from pies to cakes. As we had a garden it only seemed natural to grow our own vegetables, especially as we didn't have

'Dinner Lady Wanted', for ten hours a week, two hours a day during term-time.

much disposable income. I didn't really think about it at the time, but it was good family food, and we all took it for granted.

When the boys got a little older, I looked around for a part-time job, which would bring in some extra cash. Money was always tight, but that's not surprising, with three fast-growing lads to feed and clothe. I went to work in the local pub, where I'd been briefly before, but this time with quite a bit more knowledge about cooking. It was Sue, the landlady at that time, who encouraged me, and after working alongside her for a while, learning the ropes, I started to cook on my own. It was quite a step from cooking for a family to cooking for other people, but I enjoyed it. The food was quite simple, and a lot of it was pre-prepared, but the lasagnes and pies were all cooked from scratch. There were also some mixed grills, steaks and salads on the menu, so I was starting to be creative. This was my first introduction to catering en masse. At one point, Sue and her family went on holiday and left me on my own for three weeks. I have never been so exhausted in my life, as I was running the bar, looking after staff, cooking part-time, and also had a family to look after. When they came back from holiday they actually offered me the job of managing the pub. Although I knew the kids were all right, as George was on shifts and could look after them – or my Mum did – I decided that I wasn't seeing enough of any of my family, and that the job just wasn't possible at that stage of my life.

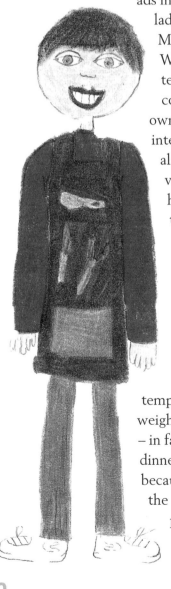

I needed a job that would fit in with the children, and started looking at the ads in the local paper. That was when my journey as a dinner lady really started, when I applied for a position at the Mount Primary School in Newark, in 1989. 'Dinner Lady Wanted', for ten hours a week, two hours a day during term-time. It sounded like the perfect part-time job, combining my love of cooking with being around for my own kids after school and during the holidays. I went for an interview, but sadly didn't get the job, which went to a girl already working in the kitchen. But they had another vacancy, as a kitchen assistant, which involved half an hour less each day. I took it, as I thought it was a foot in the door.

I started working in the kitchens for just an hour and a half each day. It was hard work – and nothing really to do with cooking at all – but I loved it. The kitchen had to be cleaned to a very high standard and I can still remember scrubbing the tiled floor on my hands and knees, washing down the paintwork as well as moving fridges and freezers and scrubbing pots and pans. It was hard labour. We sweated in the summer months as the temperatures soared and I hoped that I would lose a bit of weight, but I didn't! I worked with a fantastic bunch of girls – in fact, I don't think I've ever worked in a school where the dinner ladies haven't all had a great rapport. Perhaps it's because we're all mums together, or that we all want to do the best for the kids we're looking after. (I still meet this particular group for coffee every now and again, when I'm not gallivanting all over the country. We have remained good friends.)

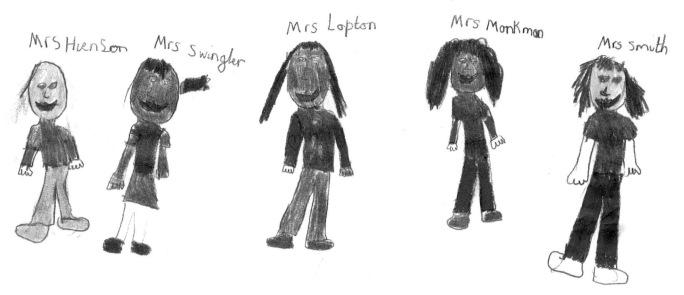

Mrs Huenson Mrs Swingler Mrs Lopton Mrs Monkman Mrs Smith

When one of the dinner ladies was off for a while, I was promoted, as my cook-supervisor, Wendy Holmes, knew how much I loved what I was doing. At first, I was given extra hours, and I made things like salads. Within a year, though, Wendy encouraged me to apply for another position that had become vacant, and so I became the assistant cook, replacing Alice, who had retired. Wendy was fantastic to me, endlessly patient and encouraging. She trained me in the ways of the school-meals system, the endless paperwork and all about what running a busy kitchen involves. From her I learned about hygiene regulations, something that every dinner lady in the land takes very seriously. I know that no school cook or kitchen assistant will go home leaving a dirty kitchen. I also learned about portion control, how to cook for the masses (the school had 200 children) and menu planning (she devised her own menus at that time, knowing from long experience what the children liked). I lapped all this up, as I was really interested, but it was the actual cooking that I adored. Our team of dinner ladies turned up every morning and put on white hats and starched pinnies to prepare good-quality meals from fresh meat and vegetables, and to make our own desserts from basic ingredients. To see the kids enjoying home-cooked British food made the lunchtime rush worth every minute.

Our team of dinner ladies turned up every morning and put on white hats and starched pinnies to prepare good-quality meals

The school-meals system was controlled centrally then, by the local councils. They would use a vegetable or meat supplier, and negotiate a price with him to supply, say, sixty schools in the area. Most of the contracts for that meat or vegetable supplier could be for three years or more, so the price would be set at the beginning. This was certainly so as far as meat was concerned; sometimes the vegetable prices would allow for fluctuation. So the buying was very regimented, but we didn't really know any better then. As long as we were getting fresh food – meat, vegetables, milk, everything as it should be – we were happy. At that time food was not high priority. The food scares and the E numbers etc. were not talked about or known about, or if they were in existence, they hadn't come into the public domain. So we may not have known where the foods were coming from, but at least we were making everything from scratch.

I was happy in my new role, and stayed there for over two years, but after a while I decided I needed a change and a new challenge. So when Wendy suggested that I apply for an assistant cook's post she'd seen advertised, at the school in the village where I lived, I thought I'd try, although I wasn't over-enthusiastic

As long as we were getting fresh food – meat, vegetables, milk, everything as it should be – we were happy.

as it was a smaller school. I filled in the forms and was given an interview, but the position went to the lady who'd been acting assistant cook at the school – yet again! So I stayed on at the Mount for another six months. When the position of cook-supervisor came up at the school in Bingham, Wendy said I should apply for it if I wanted to further my career. The acting cook-supervisor, who has since retired, but who became a very good friend, actually got the position. I must admit I was disappointed, but all was not lost. The contract manager at the time, a lady called Mabel Elias, told me that the cook-supervisor at a primary school nearby – St Peter's in East Bridgford – was soon to retire.

The interview took place with the head teacher at the time, Garth Powell, and the then chair of governors, the vicar at East Bridgford, Canon Alan Haydock. This time, I was very pleased to be told that I'd been given the position. Garth, who has since retired, still pops into the kitchen, and says that I was one of his most inspired appointments. I'm glad that I was. If I had gone to the Bingham school, the story would be completely different, and I wouldn't be where I am today.

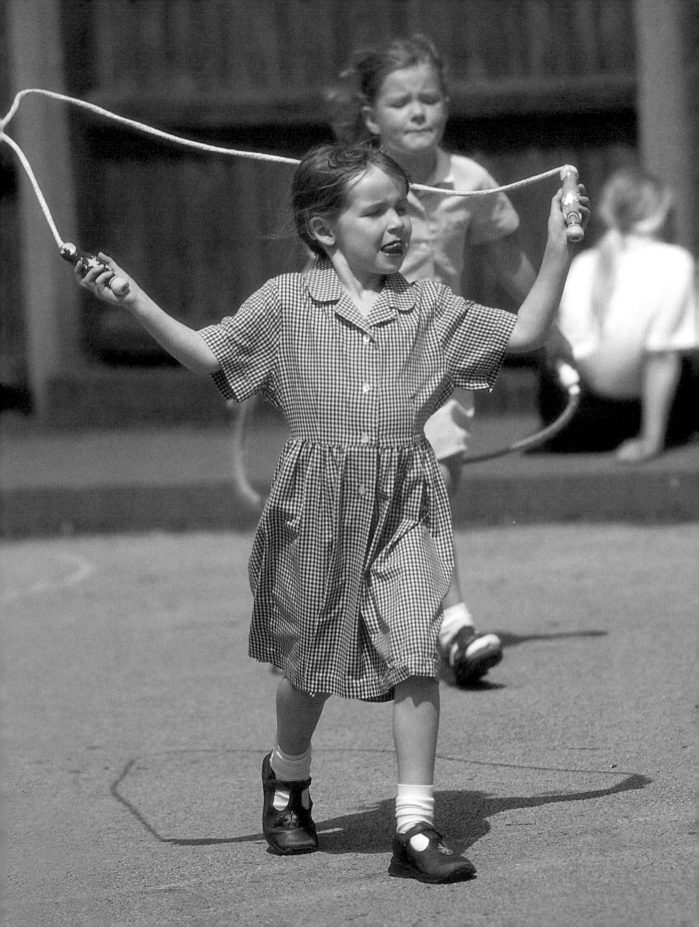

A BRIEF HISTORY OF SCHOOL DINNERS

In around 1900, there was general concern about the health of the British people. Even some fifty years after the horrors of the Industrial Revolution, child mortality was still high, living conditions were overcrowded and insanitary, and army leaders were shocked to find that many of the young men recruited for the Boer War (1899–1902) were small, undernourished and generally unfit to fight. The primary problem was poverty: wages were too low to guarantee a decent standard of living, and many children born malnourished were to remain so.

Organizations like the Salvation Army began offering cheap meals for children. The London Schools Board had established a School Dinners Association in 1889 to offer cheap, or free, school meals. With the advent of compulsory education, it had been recognized that hungry children cannot learn. By 1904 some 350 voluntary bodies were providing meals for undernourished children.

In 1906, the newly elected Liberal government passed the Education (Provision of Meals) Act to ensure that British children could grow up healthily. The act allowed Local Education Authorities (LEAs) to contribute to school canteen committees and, in certain cases, to provide free meals for the poorest children. By 1920, after a slump in numbers during World War One, over a million children were being provided with meals.

Free milk in schools was introduced in 1924 (to be withdrawn in the early 1970s by Margaret Thatcher, 'Milk Snatcher'). By 1940, government was paying 95 per cent of the cost of meals, and recommendations on nutritional content, staffing levels and organization of service were introduced. The Education Act of 1944 made compulsory what had previously been performed by LEAs on a voluntary basis: every child in a maintained school had to be provided with a meal. 1.8 million children were now taking school meals. By 1947, the full cost of school meals was met by government.

During the 1950s, the price of school meals went up gradually (from 6d to 1/-, or double). In 1967, though, the 100 per cent governmental grant for school expenditure was withdrawn. In 1978, a government white paper on public expenditure estimated the cost of producing school meals at £380 million, and targeted a reduction to £190 million. This immediately reduced the quality of the meals and service provided, and convenience meals began to be commonplace. At the same time, the dreaded cafeteria was introduced into secondary schools. And then in 1980 the new Education Act gave LEAs the power to axe the school meals service (see page 40). The era of the processed dinner had begun.

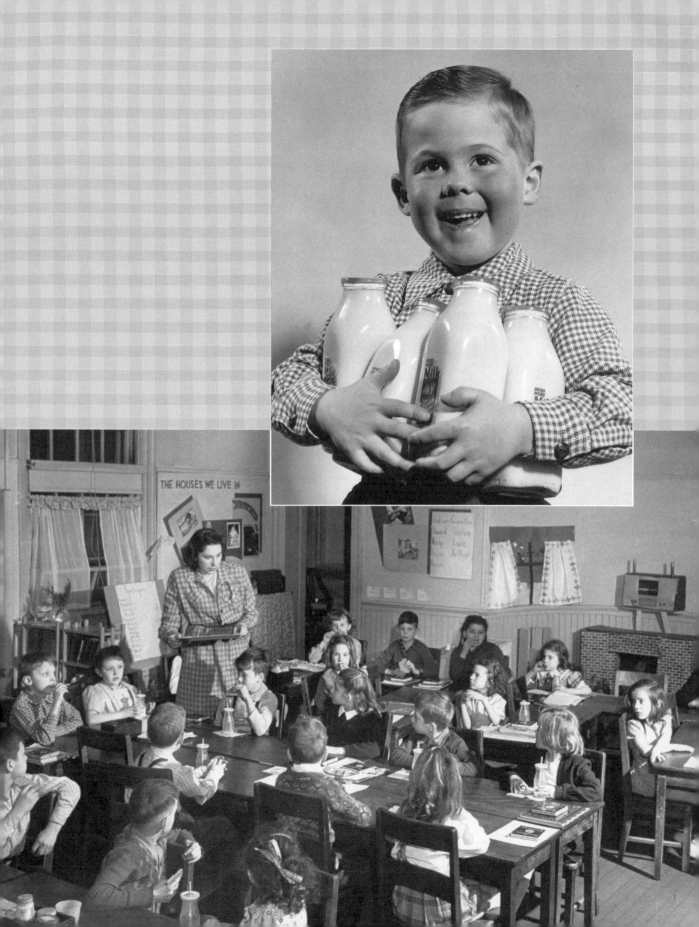

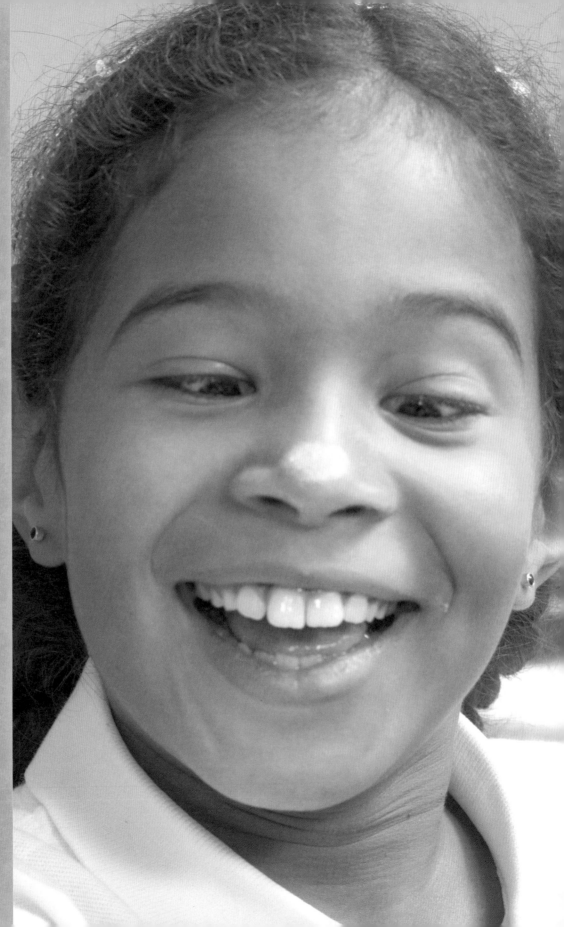

WHEN I FIRST STARTED at St Peter's in 1992 I found a very streamlined operation, much like it had been in Newark, but with only about seventy pupils taking lunch each day out of a possible 200 or so (the rest brought in packed lunches). My job as cook-supervisor involved the general management of the school kitchen, including cooking, cleaning and the serving of meals. I was also responsible for the day-to-day running of all the kitchen equipment, and making sure the school kitchen ran smoothly. On a daily basis I had to:

- Compile the staff rotas and supervise all kitchen staff.

- Do all the administration work in connection with catering, including menu planning etc., food ordering, stock control, costing and the maintenance of staff record sheets and reports as required.

- Conduct risk assessments.

- Cook all school meals with help from the kitchen staff.

- Maintain strict adherence to health & safety and hygiene regulations.

- Manage all kitchen staff.

- Conduct the induction programme for new staff.

The retiring cook-supervisor had run a tight, even regimented ship, but as with everything in life, we all have our own ways of doing things. Wendy had let me go to St Peter's before my predecessor retired to see how everything operated before I officially started, as each kitchen is individual. I can remember feeling very nervous, but I wanted to introduce myself to the rest of the kitchen staff. It was then that I met Christine Derry, the kitchen assistant. She was very quiet, one of those people who just got on with the job in hand and left at the end of the day.

On my first official morning at St Peter's I had arrived early, and set to getting everything prepared for lunch, which meant peeling the carrots and potatoes and getting the meat ready for the oven. When Christine arrived, she looked at me, then around the kitchen, and asked what we were cooking for lunch as there were no pots in the sink. I actually hadn't done much work, for to me prepping seventy meals from doing over 200, as in Newark, was a holiday. I later found out that the former cook would rarely say 'good morning' to Christine. All she sometimes got was a bark of 'windows!' or 'pans!' – an order for her to get polishing or scrubbing. (In those days cleanliness really was next to godliness.) And so polishing and scrubbing was all Christine did from the moment she arrived until two hours later. I think my motto of 'clean as you go' cemented our friendship for ever. She is still the most gentle person I have ever met, but, some fourteen years later, she is now in charge of the kitchen at St Peter's. She's come a long way, because when I first started, she couldn't – and wouldn't – do anything so far as cooking was concerned. I remember the first time I asked her to roll pastry out, and she said she didn't know how. I told her not to be so silly, and gave her a few pointers. Basically what I did was leave her to get on with it and, of course, she's now a dab hand at pastry. She's a really good person, and a very talented one, able to take most things I throw at her (well, not literally).

There were three of us in the kitchen then. Lynn came in a lot later in the morning than Christine and I to help with the setting out of the dining hall, and washing the pots. She worked only a few hours a week, but this suited her. She lived on the RAF base very near to us, where many of the mums wanted a few hours' work a week. Unfortunately, her husband was soon posted abroad and we lost her. But then Christine's sister, Alison Ellis, came to work for me, and has been at St Peter's ever since. As far

... to me prepping seventy meals from doing 200, as in Newark, was a holiday.

as the food was concerned at that time, we were cooking a simple menu of fresh meat and vegetables and a home-made sweet. I was working in the ways I'd been taught, which suited all of us, including the council and the head (who was due to retire), and I generally went home satisfied that I had done a good job of providing the kids with a tasty lunch. In fact, we raised the number of children who wanted to stay for dinner from seventy-five to ninety in no time at all, so we must have been doing something right.

For the next five years or so, everything continued happily, and we continued to increase the numbers of children staying for school dinners (important to us

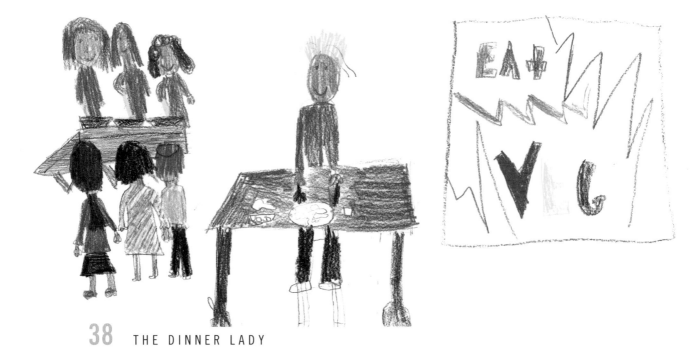

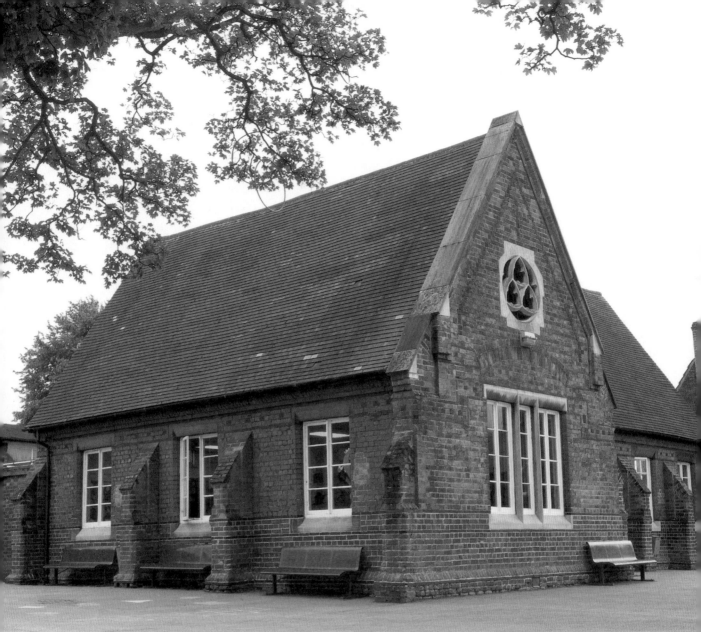

because it meant that our hours in the kitchen were increased). It's a good thing work was going so well because my personal life suffered a major blow when George was involved in a horrific car accident in December 1996. He had broken all the ribs on his right side, puncturing his lung twice, and I was told he had a 10 per cent chance of survival. The fact that he was so fit contributed, so I was told, to saving his life, but he was to be off work until the summer, and my life went on hold too for several months. But when I came back to school, my job was still waiting for me and so were my friends. Any dinner lady reading this book will recognize this, knowing about the friendships that exist within the kitchen environment.

Declining Standards

THE PEOPLE WHO CREATED the welfare state fully understood the role of the school meals service, seeing it as crucial in the fight against poverty and malnutrition. But the 1980 Education Act, nearly forty years after the founding of the welfare state, was to downgrade school meals to being non-essential. In other words, the act gave LEAs (Local Education Authorities) the power to axe the school meals service, thereby removing the duty to provide a midday meal that was 'suitable in all respects as the main meal of the day', something that had been introduced as long before as 1944. The act also got rid of the minimum nutritional standards that controlled the quality of school meals and the fixed price 'national charge'.

There were now only two statutory requirements: first, that LEAs must ensure that children whose parents receive supplementary benefit or family income support receive a free meal; and second, that facilities must be provided for pupils who bring their own food. As a direct result of this act, the number of children taking school meals in primary schools dropped to 41.7 per cent, and 53.4 per cent in secondary schools – and this after it had been recorded that 60 per cent of all schoolchildren were taking school dinners some three years earlier. Some councils in England even voted to discontinue the school meals service altogether.

... contractors knew they could rely on the goodwill of dinner ladies, who would always try, against all odds, to ensure that their children ate well.

St Peter's was unaffected for a while, as were a lot of other schools around the country, because contractors knew they could rely on the goodwill of dinner ladies, who would always try, against all odds, to ensure that their children ate well. And Nottinghamshire Council continued to provide a school meals service. However, in 1996, something called Compulsory Competitive Tendering hit the school meals service in Nottinghamshire and elsewhere. CCT was a requirement for public agencies such as local authorities to put certain services out to competitive tender. Managers are required to give the work to the contractor who best meets specified criteria, in particular, cost reduction. Initially introduced into hospitals in 1983 and extended to local government by the Local Government Act of 1988, it primarily affected services such as cleaning, catering and laundry in hospitals and schools, refuse collection, and so on. Although many contracts remained 'in-house', the process of tendering allowed managers to alter employment practices and, often, terms and conditions of employment. In other words, in most cases, the poorly paid became even poorer.

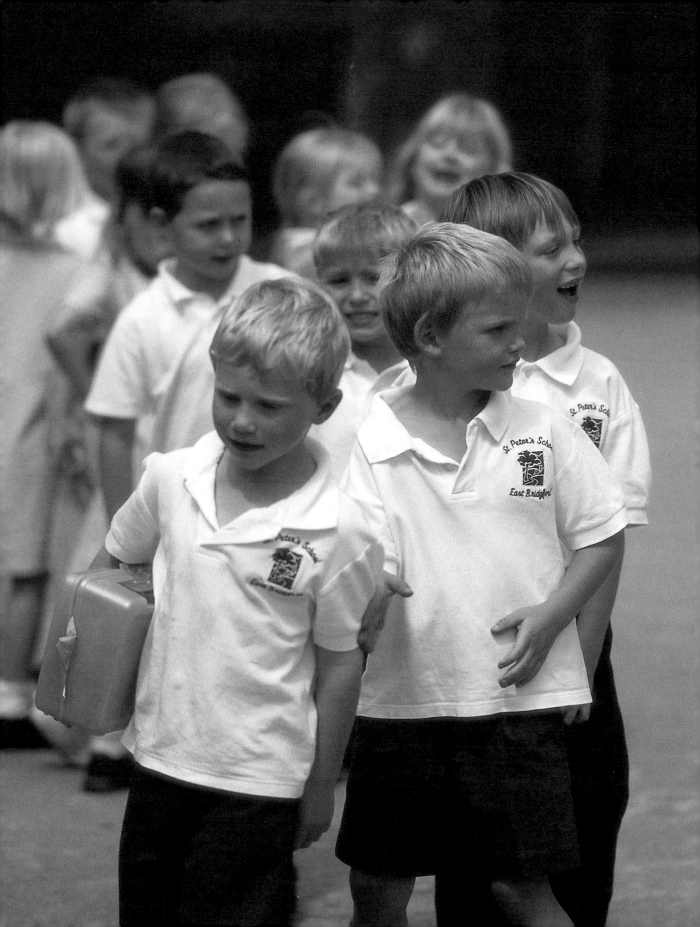

What happened in our case was that the council walked into our kitchens, took out all of our equipment, reduced our hours and brought in pre-prepared 'food'. We didn't need the equipment any more, they said, because all the food would come in ready for use. And because the food was coming in packets, all we dinner ladies needed was the ability to use a pair of scissors. Cutting open a packet of pastry mix doesn't need much skill, and certainly doesn't involve much time – so they cut back on actual numbers of dinner ladies, and on their hours of work. I had been working thirty hours a week by then, but these were cut back to twenty-eight, and all the other ladies in the kitchen lost hours as well.

They called this CCT process 'best value'. One wonders for whom – for the children, for their parents, or for the school? – but all too soon it became apparent that 'best value' unfortunately meant the cheapest. The advantages of CCT – if you can call them that – are that councils get to see who is in the marketplace, what is available in the way of services, and what difference there is in costs. But the problem with CCT – and this 'one' problem considerably outweighs the advantages – is that prices are constantly driven downwards, which means that to be competitive contractors constantly strive to cut corners and reduce services to stay within budget. This usually meant the loss of jobs, but it also meant that producers – farmers and growers – were having constantly to reduce *their* costs to remain within the marketplace.

What CCT meant as far as we were concerned in the St Peter's kitchen was that the quality of the food deteriorated. Under CCT, there were no mandatory nutritional standards. Although you could, at a push, call us fortunate in

Nottinghamshire, because we still had a school meals service of sorts, we also had people at the top who obviously 'knew best'. We dinner ladies knew better, though. Vegetables arrived almost any way you liked them, sliced, diced and bagged up in advance so that a considerable proportion of the nutrients had completely vanished by the time they were cooked. It must also have been cheaper for them to send pre-prepared vegetables than to service the machinery that did the job for us. Our potato 'Rumbler' (the industrial peeler) was replaced with a constant supply of ready-quartered spuds, preserved in a slimy whitening agent that was supposed to keep them looking nice. But in reality this had a strong chemical smell that we could never entirely wash off, even when we put in an extra hour to do so.

The meat would be frozen: what they call 'free-flow mince' (because it flowed 'freely' out of the packet), and as we opened the packets with scissors, the stench was awful. A shepherd's pie, for instance, would consist of this mince (probably from eleven different cows from eleven different countries), frozen chopped carrots, ready-diced onions, and not those unpleasant potatoes, but dried potato. (You must remember that it would take at least twenty minutes to boil those potatoes, and we didn't have those hours in the kitchen.) As a result, our job became

Our job became more like that of an assembly line, bringing things together rather than cooking

more like that of an assembly line, bringing things together rather than cooking, and we had nothing at our disposal, apart from gravy browning or Marmite, to make the dish *taste* nice (the prerequisite of *anything* we eat, I would have thought). Our home-made desserts were replaced with packets of sponge mix, packets of pastry mix, packets of crumble mix, anything-you-like mix. All we had to do was scissor open the package, get out measuring jugs, pour in the required amount of water, and mix. This wasn't real food; this was the start of an era of cheap processed muck, and it was marching across the country.

There were also all these 'shaped' processed foods designed for children. A despairing primary head was once quoted in a paper as saying, 'The children don't ask me what they are having for lunch any more. They ask me what *shape* they are having. They have learned they can't tell the difference on the basis of texture or taste.' At St Peter's we used to be sent in things like chicken nuggets, chicken teddies, turkey twizzlers, pork hippos and fishysauruses, which were all highly processed foods. For instance, the fish content of the latter (shaped like whales) was fairly minimal, the rest being rusk, dextrose, starch, additives and the breadcrumb coating. The pork hippos were the greatest disaster. After they had been baking for the suggested time, Christine opened the oven, and the smell that hit us was appalling. Without even thinking, I threw them all in the bin, and made something else very quickly. That was the only time I ever served a school dinner late.

And then the local authority started to dictate the menus weeks in advance. At the beginning of my time at St Peter's we were on 'Family Service', which meant we 'cooked' and served one set meal per day. We would get this six-week rolling menu coming from someone up high who didn't have a clue about what the children liked and disliked at our school. *We* knew on the ground, but no one thought to ask us. So when we were forced to serve shepherd's pie on Monday, chicken nuggets on Tuesday, frozen pizzas (we could assemble those, but on a frozen base, obviously), and processed this and that for the rest of the week, we were faced with a load of hungry and miserable children – and lots of unemptied plates. Because

The pork hippos were the greatest disaster.

the quality of the packet pastries and sponges was so poor (many of us refused to work with the pastry, saying it was like concrete), I and many other dinner ladies would make our own. This would obviously cost extra in cash terms, and indeed time, and we wouldn't get any more money in wages for this. The powers that be must have realized that most dinner ladies would not want to serve complete swill to the children, and so they were perhaps relying on our goodwill. It was a dreadful situation.

The ladies in my kitchen were demoralized, de-skilled and because of the new pre-prepared menus and foods, their hours were cut. We used to have to go to cook-supervisors' meetings, probably once a term, and I can remember one cook saying she was only going to stick her time out until she retired. Others were sick and tired of the way they had been treated, but we all continued to work bloody hard. We were troopers. We dubbed ourselves the 'can-do ladies' and joked that we could still do anything, with not a lot. And then throughout the county (and probably the whole country), as dinner ladies left, through demoralization or simply retirement, the local authorities started to bring in regeneration ovens. These marked one further step down the ladder, because everything, and I mean everything, was already done for you. The food came into these schools frozen in foil containers, and all they had to do was heat it through in the oven and then serve it – rather like microwave-oven meals today. To me this was appalling: at least before dinner ladies had played some part, however minimal, in putting the food together. With regeneration ovens, they had no hand whatsoever in what was being served, what it looked like or what it tasted like.

As the nutritional value of what we served plummeted, the kids were being stuffed with artificial junk. We were told it was more cost-effective to produce school dinners this way, but to whom? All I knew was that the children were paying the price. For what it was worth, I thought that the system was dangerously misguided, putting profit before health and nutrition. What the children ate seemed to be at the bottom of the list of priorities, and we all know how important it is to feed children properly. If dinner ladies were worried about the effect it would have on the kids, why wasn't anybody else?

WHEN I WAS GROWING UP – which wasn't all *that* long ago – there wasn't such a thing as food specially aimed at children. My mum, and her mum before her, cooked good, honest, plain English food such as roasts and casseroles, with the occasional beans on toast or a fry-up. We ate vegetables in season, Mum made cakes or biscuits for my brother and I when we came home from school, and we might have a treat of fish and chips (with tomato sauce and vinegar, of course) on a Friday night now and again. We children ate what the adults ate, and didn't think about it, didn't expect anything else.

Today, however, all that has changed, and children's food has become big business. Freezer cabinets and supermarket shelves are stuffed with processed foods with bright and breezy packaging 'designed' for kids. Television adverts, often featuring popular real-life or fictional stars, sell these foods to young and naive customers. Pubs and popular restaurant chains have children's menus that offer 'everything with chips'. These chips, sausages, burgers, fish fingers, chicken nuggets and a multitude of other 'child-friendly', often bizarrely shaped foods are also stuffed full of additives, such as colourings, flavourings, preservatives and bulking additives, as well as sugar, salt and fat. Can these foods really be good for our children? I think not. There are a few facts below that might enlighten you as to what your children are actually eating.

Up to one year, babies are protected from all those horrors. In the UK there are strict laws that control what can and cannot be added to infant formulas and baby foods. These rules help protect babies from ingesting additives that their immature livers and kidneys cannot cope with. But after a year, the laws vanish, and the one-year-old baby can then eat the same as adults. If we were still eating the healthy basic meals of our childhoods, we wouldn't have to worry at all. But we're not: nowadays all of us are offered an array of heavily processed foods, and children are offered those 'special' foods packed with the additives the law forbids in foods for babies. How can a mere one-year-old cope with that?

It's frightening to me, because children, more than any other group, are 'what they eat', and what they eat is absolutely vital because they are growing and developing so rapidly. They need honest, good foods with nutrients that will build bones and develop the brain. They don't need to be stuffed full of additives, sugar and salt, all of which can lead to disease now and in the future. We are only just beginning to realize how important it is for the diet to be good

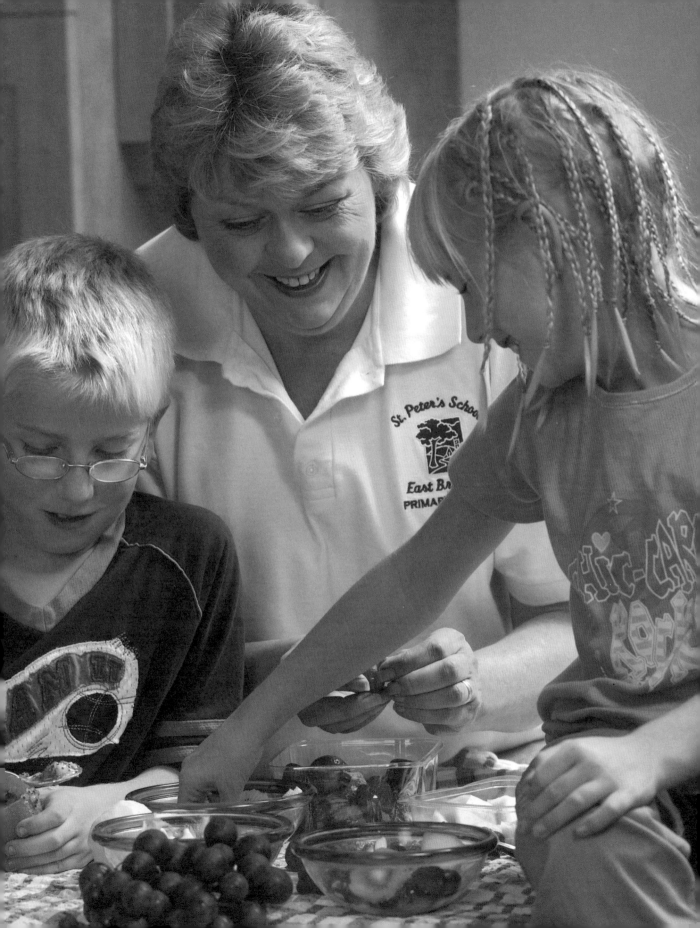

when children are young. As with obesity, the initial damage can be done when a child is under ten, and the disease process set in train at that time can emerge later on in life.

The organic baby-food company Organix carried out a recent survey, testing 365 children's foods for additives – colourings, flavourings, preservatives, sugar, salt, fat, etc. – and the results were horrifying. The worst offenders were, as you might expect, sweets, cereal bars, crisps, breakfast cereals, children's desserts and drinks, and frozen beefburgers. The survey found no less than an average of five additives per children's food tested.

Colourings

Many colourings used in this country were originally derived from coal tar (now made synthetically) and they have been linked to hyperactivity and asthma in some children. The survey found that one-third of the foods tested contained colourings. One piece of confectionery alone contained no fewer than seven!

Flavourings

75 per cent of the children's foods tested contained artificial flavourings. These too can cause allergy. And if food needs disguising to make it taste good, wouldn't you do better without it?

Preservatives

25 per cent of the children's foods tested contained preservatives. Many of these (E numbers 200–285) are known to trigger side effects, including allergy and hyperactivity, in children. And, another take on preservatives, they are actually there to keep food 'fresh' long after it should have gone stale …

Bulking additives

Mostly starch and sugar based, these are added to children's processed foods to bulk them out, and as a result they form a good proportion of many foods. These 'empty calories' supply energy, of course, but no nutrients.

Sugar

The Organix survey had difficulty, due to poor labelling, in working out the precise sugar content of sweet foods. On average, though, in the foods tested, it was almost 70 per cent, which is horrifying. Sugar is a carbohydrate, but unlike other carbs, such as starches (vegetables, fruit, pulses and grains), it is 'empty' of all goodness and contains only calories. All the sugars that we eat – sucrose (refined white sugar), fructose (fruit), lactose (milk) etc. – are potentially harmful in general terms, particularly as regards obesity, but even more so dentally.

Sugar reacts with the bacteria and plaque that occur naturally in the mouth to create acid. This acid then eats into the enamel of teeth and causes decay. Much dental damage can be done very early, as many parents get their toddlers off to sleep with a bottle of juice or, worse still, a dummy dipped in honey. This means that the mouth is receiving extra sugar for a long time, overnight even. Most dentists actually advise that if any sweet thing is to be eaten – by child or adult – it should be in one fell swoop. Frequency of sugar intake is the most potentially damaging, for every time sugar comes in touch with plaque, the acid produced will stay on the teeth (and have its way on the enamel) for up to twenty minutes (unless naturally washed off by saliva or brushed off with toothpaste). To illustrate the point, one campaigning dentist suggested that it was better for a child to eat one whole packet of boiled sweets in one go than to suck those sweets individually throughout the day. Even the most sweet-loving child would find that difficult, I think!

Babies naturally like sweet flavours, as breast milk itself is sweet. This liking, very mistakenly, is catered for by manufacturers of babies' and children's drinks, foods and medicines. Many infant fruit drinks are advertised as packed with goodness and vitamin C, but they are also packed with sugar. The same is true of the drinks, fizzy and still, produced for older children. In fact, one day at St Peter's, we had a little demonstration. We soaked teeth (supplied by a dentist parent) in cola, lemon juice and water – and the results, very visual, left our nine-year-olds in little doubt about the impact of sweet sugary drinks on their own gnashers!

Many snack foods aimed at children – and backed by massive advertising – contain refined sugar. The obvious culprits are cakes, biscuits, jams and fruits canned in syrup. Sweetened breakfast cereals are a particular case in point, and their role in diet-related disease was targeted by MPs in a health select committee report on obesity in early 2004. In response, one manufacturer produced reduced-sugar breakfast cereals, but the sugar content is still comparatively high. (Many cereals popular with children are also quite high in salt.) Even so-called 'health' cereals sometimes have high levels of sugar. Less refined cereals, such as Weetabix, Shredded Wheat and oats, contain much less sugar and salt.

Less obvious culprits are the foods containing 'hidden' sugars, in foods we think of as sugar-free, because they are 'savoury'. They include bread, canned tomato soup (until recently one brand contained 5.2g sugar per 100g), tomato ketchup, canned peas, beans and spaghetti, and even corned beef! (Always look at the label: if a sugar is high on the list of ingredients, the product contains a high level of sugar.) Perhaps the most disturbing way in which sugar is used is in children's medicines – to make them more 'palatable' (and to make them last longer, for sugar is a preservative). A large number of liquid antibiotics, vitamins, cough mixtures and tranquillizers use a base of sugar syrup. A survey in the 1980s found that no fewer than 21 out of 22 liquid antibiotics contained sugar.

Children who snack all day on processed foods that contain sugar (and potato crisps and some French fries contain sugar as well as salt) will be endangering their teeth quite considerably. Although a nationwide survey in 2004 showed that older children, those between eight and fifteen, had fewer fillings than was the case twenty years earlier, there had been no similar improvement for five-year-olds. New figures showed that the average five-year-old in large parts of the country had three teeth that were rotten or filled, and the number of younger children with cavities fell by only 1 per cent between 1983 and 2003 to 40 per cent, despite the widespread introduction of fluoride toothpaste during that time. And the 2003 Dental Health Survey of more than 12,000 children found that only 59 per cent of English five-year-olds were free of decay, despite a target of 70 per cent.

But children who snack all day on foods high in sugar are also endangering their general health. All carbohydrates, of which sugar is one, supply energy, a necessity for all of us, particularly growing children. If a child is eating only highly refined sugary foods, he is not only *not* eating good food, but he is eating food that will satisfy him in energy terms for a very short space of time. The glycaemic index (used widely by diabetes sufferers) defines foods as healthy or less healthy according to the rate at which they are converted into blood sugar.

Refined sugary foods, those that are high on the index, are rapidly converted, which leads to body and mood highs and lows, and these are linked with behavioural and metabolic abnormalities, and with diabetes

Children who snack all day on foods high in sugar are also endangering their general health.

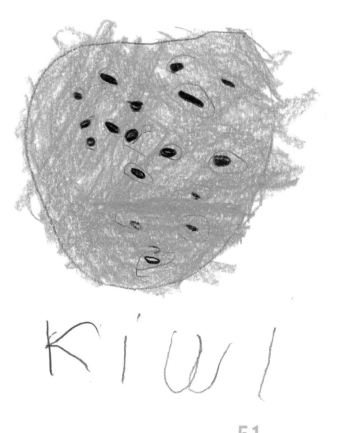

and obesity. Less refined or unrefined carbohydrates would satisfy a child for much longer, and to a far higher nutritional standard (Shredded Wheat and Weetabix in preference to sweeter cereals, although fresh fruit would be good too for breakfast).

The idea that five-year-olds have to be sedated by dentists to have bad teeth extracted is bad enough, but what is even worse in a dental sense is that the decay could affect both the second teeth – the teeth we keep for life – and jaw formation. However, what is worst of all is the possibility that some children who are eating a refined sugary diet are likely to not be getting sufficient nutrients for their needs.

Shocking stuff, but we have to be practical about it. Sugar and sugary foods exist, and children like them. So, how to cut down on their intake? The most important thing to me, obviously, is for parents to avoid buying manufactured foods with hidden sugars as far as possible, and to choose, cook and serve fresh foods. If you make cakes and biscuits at home, at least you will know how much sugar is in them (and you're not going to do that very often anyway). Do obvious things like banning the sugar bowl, and not over-sweetening stewed fruit and other dishes. Perhaps make savoury dishes more attractive than sweet dishes. Meals don't have to include a sweet dish – you could serve a starter and main course instead of a main course and pudding, or make it a habit just to offer fruit. Children love puddings, though, and all contain sugar, but you can cut the sugar content down gradually. That's what I have done at St Peter's – and in the recipes at the end of the book – and I haven't had any complaints so far. As for the sweets question, that's quite difficult. A total ban would achieve the opposite effect, making sweets more desirable. If the child were allowed sweets once a week, say, he or she wouldn't feel deprived, and would actually have something to look forward to. It's worth a try, anyway …

If the child were allowed sweets once a week, say, he or she wouldn't feel deprived, and would actually have something to look forward to.

Salt

A headline in the *Daily Mail* of 13 September 2004 read 'How millions are being "poisoned" by too much salt'. In the article, the Food Standards Agency warned that the maximum recommended safe limit of salt for adults – 5ml or 1 teaspoon (6g) per day, half that for small children – was being exceeded regularly by up to 26 million people, some 2.3 million of them consuming up to 18g per day (about 3 $1/2$ heaped teaspoons). The pressure group that had originally raised the issue – Consensus Action on Salt and Health or CASH (based at St George's Hospital in London) – pointed out that because of this excess, thousands were dying prematurely per annum of stroke and heart disease.

We all need a certain proportion of salt, for our bodies naturally contain it (blood is salty, as are sweat and tears), and too little salt causes low blood

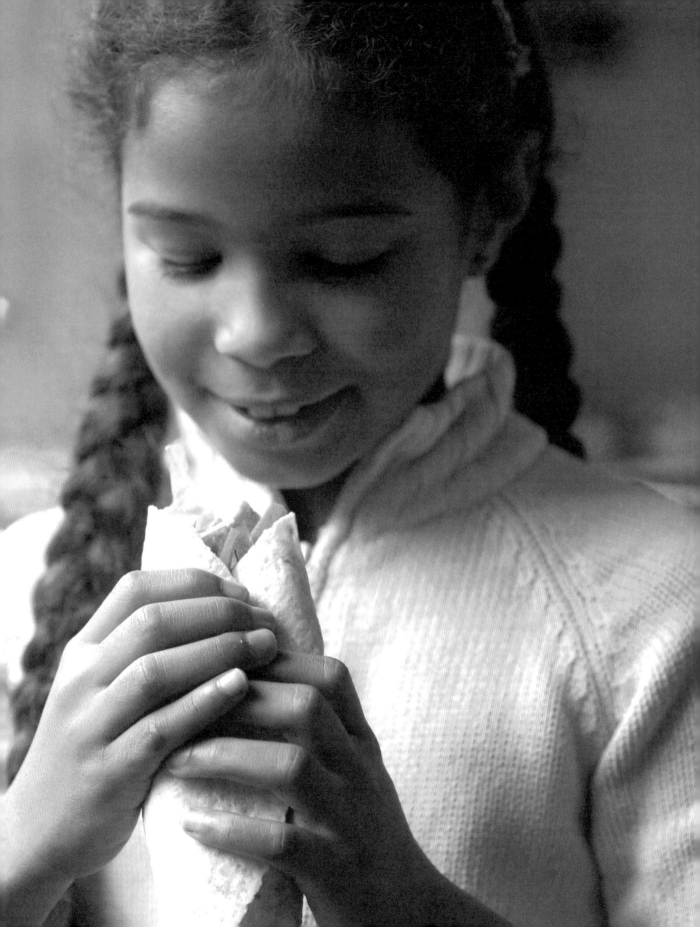

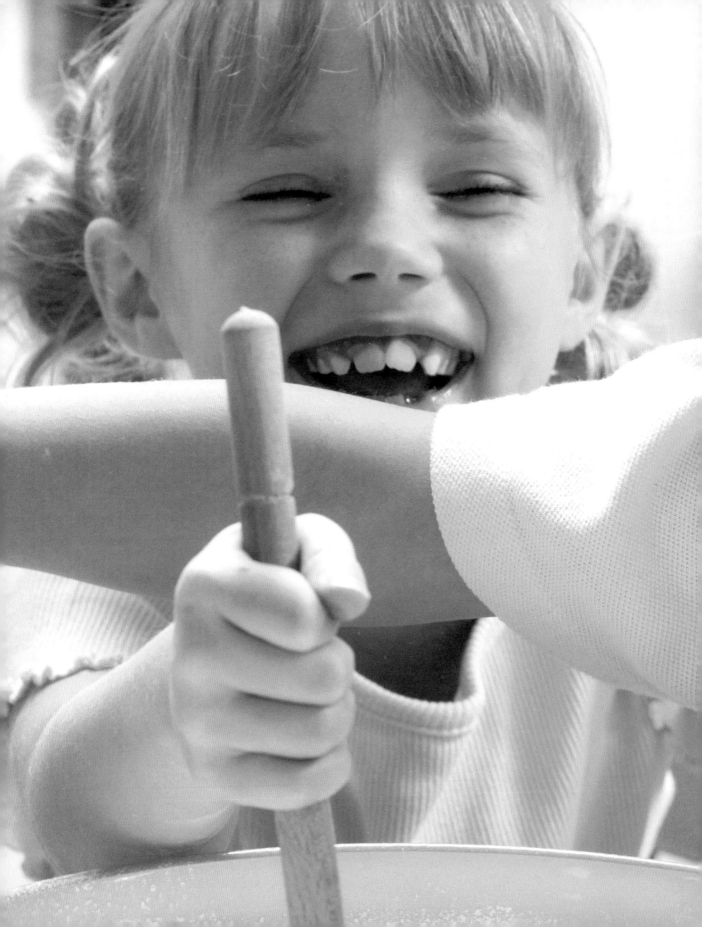

pressure and dizziness. But too much salt in the diet *raises* blood pressure, which is far more dangerous. As salt levels in the blood go up, water is attracted into the blood from the muscles and organs to dilute it. The more fluid that is carried in the blood, the harder the heart has to work to pump the same amount round the body. This is what high blood pressure (HBP) is, and in adults it leads to strokes, heart attacks, the swelling of oedema, and certain cancers. Professor Graham MacGregor of CASH says that people who eat too much salt can have 1.5 litres (no less than 2 ³/₄ pints) of extra fluid sloshing around in their veins. As the annual cost of NHS drugs to reduce HBP is around £840 million, nearly 15 per cent of the total cost of primary care, no wonder the government is anxious to encourage us to eat less salt. (I'm not sure, though, about the effectiveness of Sid the Slug…)

However, that recommended maximum level of salt is very difficult to stick to. It is not much use stopping adding salt at the side of the plate (although it is a great start), as salt is a component of so many things we eat. As with sugar, it is added to many processed foods, and there are some horrifying statistics, prime among them the fact that 80 per cent of the salt we eat is 'hidden' salt. CASH found that a bowlful of one supermarket breakfast cereal – sold as a 'health' food – contained 1.8g salt, almost 30 per cent of the daily requirement. Another supermarket's farmhouse loaf contained 1g of salt in every slice, making it '70 per cent as salty as the ocean', to quote a newspaper journalist. More obvious salt-laden foods were sausages, pizzas, fishcakes, baked beans, canned soups, cooking sauces and pork pies. CASH said that anyone living for a day on such foods would get about 25g salt, which is much more than the maximum recommended by the Food Standards Agency.

If salt is bad for adults, it is worse for children.

If salt is bad for adults, it is worse for children. Babies probably are born with a taste for salty things, although it is not so strong as that for sweet things. But additional salt should always be avoided in babies' foods, as their systems cannot cope and they cannot excrete it, and the same applies for toddlers and older children. They should not be encouraged to develop a taste for highly salty foods. The irony is that the more salt there is in food, the more the body tolerates it and the more it wants. The more salt children (and adults) eat, the thirstier they get – which can lead to an increase in soft drinks (and thus sugar consumption). It's a vicious circle.

Today's children are estimated to be eating more than twice the recommended maximum intake of around 3g salt for those aged four to six, and 5g for seven to elevens, 6g for elevens and over. The Organix survey mentioned above found that just a couple of servings a day of most processed children's foods would take them over those levels. Just 20g of some savoury snacks – crisps, say – would provide a child with 50–70 per cent of the recommended maximum intake of salt for the day. To quote Professor Graham MacGregor again: 'Salt is a chronic long-term toxin which slowly raises blood pressure from childhood onwards so that as people reach middle and old age they are at ever-increasing risk of death or disability.' If too much salt in childhood can lead to disease in adulthood, isn't this persuasion enough towards feeding our children more carefully?

The best way to avoid too much salt is to eat healthily, sticking to fresh and freshly cooked food, and to avoid processed foods and ready meals. If this is not possible, either wholly or in part, always read the labels carefully. The higher the salt or sodium content is in the listing, the more salt there is. And another thing to watch: sodium is often quoted instead of salt, because it sounds like less. To estimate the salt, you need to multiply the sodium figure by 2.5, so suddenly the 2.2g of sodium is transformed into 5.5g salt (nearly a day's recommended maximum) – quite a difference! Ban the salt cellar on the table, and use less while cooking – which can mean that you actually recognize and appreciate the natural flavour of your foods more. Adding herbs and spices to foods creates flavour, so that the need for saltiness is reduced. Just tucking a couple of sprigs of fresh or dried thyme into a meat stew creates a 'savouriness'.

Fat and obesity

Some types of fat are necessary for the body, and especially for children's bodies, as fats are important during periods of growth. They also help in the absorption of the fat-soluble vitamins A, D, E and K. These necessary fats are mainly monounsaturated and polyunsaturated, and are found in seeds, grains, vegetable oils and soft margarines. Only a very small quantity of these fats is needed – some 1–2 per cent of the energy intake of the diet. Fats that are less desirable are the saturated fats, and these are found in animal fats in meat (in beef, lamb, pork, suet, lard and dripping); in dairy products such as milk, butter and cheese; in hard margarine and some vegetable oils (such as coconut and palm oils). Small proportions of these are required in the diet because of the necessary protein they contain (meat, milk and cheese, for instance). Saturated fats are also found in many bought foods such as cakes, biscuits, pastries, chocolate and ready meals.

Some types of fat are necessary for children's bodies.

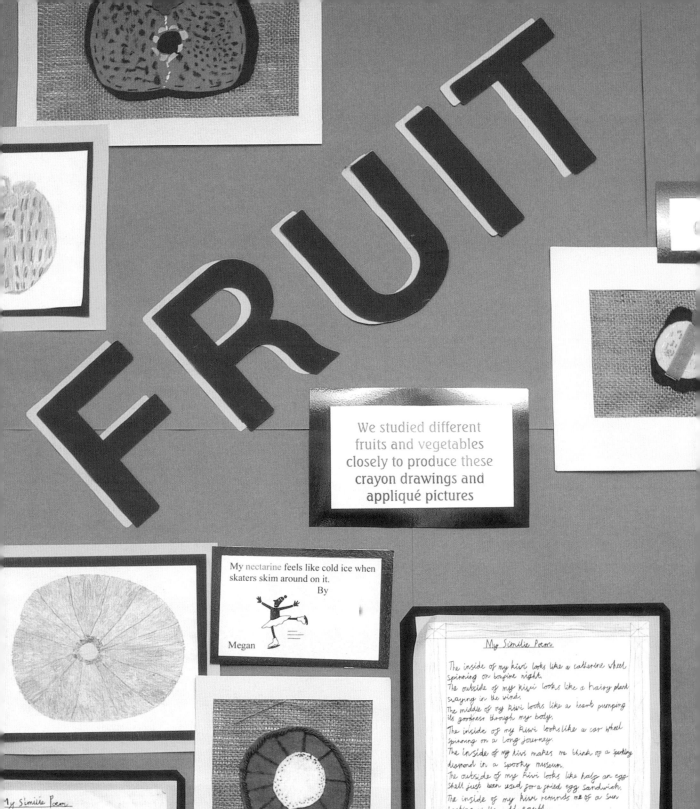

FRUIT

We studied different fruits and vegetables closely to produce these crayon drawings and appliqué pictures

My nectarine feels like cold ice when skaters skim around on it.

By

Megan

My Similie Poem

The inside of my kiwi looks like a catherine wheel spinning on bonfire night.
The outside of my kiwi looks like a hairy plant swaying in the wind.
The middle of my kiwi looks like a heart pumping its goodness through my body.
The inside of my kiwi looks like a car wheel spinning on a long journey.
The inside of my kiwi makes me think of a sparkling diamond in a spooky museum.
The outside of my kiwi looks like half an egg shell just been used for a fried egg sandwich.
The inside of my kiwi reminds me of a sun heating up the cold earth.
The inside of kiwi feels like a bar of soap ready to be used, yet worn out.

My Similie Poem

...to looks like a butterfly flapping it's wings

...feels like a snail slivering slowly across the

...reminds me of a dark damp cave by the
... side, where the waves crash like thunder.

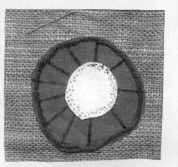

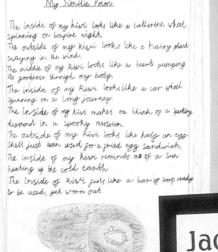

Jack
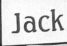

Saturated and polyunsaturated or monounsaturated fats contain the same amount of calories – how the energy value of a food is measured – but saturated fats affect blood cholesterol very much more. Cholesterol is a substance manufactured by and naturally present in the body, but it is also found in many other animal tissues, those that we eat. High levels of cholesterol in the blood, which could be a result of eating too much saturated fat, have become associated with an increased risk of heart disease as a result of fat layers forming on the walls of arteries (atherosclerosis). Some children – a few as young as eleven – have been found to have abnormally high deposits from cholesterol consumption, which makes them vulnerable to early heart disease in adulthood.

Fat babies were once thought to be the most healthy and 'bonny', but in fact were probably destined to become fat children and fat adults. Overfeeding or giving solid foods too early would have been a major reason, but what their mothers probably didn't know was that fat cells were being created and established. Research has shown that when a growing baby or child becomes too fat, the cells in his body that hold fat will increase in number as well as size. This means that he will carry those extra fat cells for the rest of his life, and fat cells demand to be filled. This is why many overweight children – and adults – find it so difficult to lose weight.

During and after World War Two, Britons were famously thought to be at their healthiest, because of rationing and a necessarily limited diet.

In Britain, we are currently going through an epidemic of childhood obesity. Between 1984 and 1994, obesity in children apparently rose alarmingly, and the link began to be made with the first cases of type-2 diabetes among teenagers in the UK. (Previously diabetes was a 'late onset' disease, traditionally affecting only adults.) According to official figures from the Office of National Statistics (ONS) in 2004, 1 in 7 fifteen-year-olds and 1 in 12 six-year-olds were obese; obesity had risen by three-fifths in boys and two-fifths in girls since 1995. In June 2004, the Pre-School Learning Alliance pointed to statistics predicting that, under current trends, more than 40 per cent of the UK population could be obese within a generation. And obesity itself is thought to be responsible for 31,000 premature deaths each year.

During and after World War Two, Britons were famously thought to be at their healthiest, because of rationing and a necessarily limited diet. A recent study comparing the weight and growth of school pupils fed on a 1940s diet with those (the same age group and at the same school) fed on a contemporary menu rich in junk food, outlines where the obesity today is originating.

Professor Philip James, head of global think-tank the International Obesity Task Force, said children in the 1940s – who were considered very healthy – consumed about 1800 calories daily, roughly the amount required for a growing eight-year-old, according to nutritional guidelines. The equivalent child today, because of the typical diet of crisps, hamburgers and chocolate, consumes more than 3000 calories a day – which is actually nearer the recommended daily calorie requirement of a grown man. (The results observed in this particular study were astounding. The 'wartime' children grew an inch in an eight-week period, without putting on a single extra pound in weight; the children on the modern diet neither lost weight nor grew so dramatically. Upward rather than outward is surely the better option.)

There are many reasons for this growth in childhood obesity. Food is much more widely available now in general than in the 1940s, but we have also

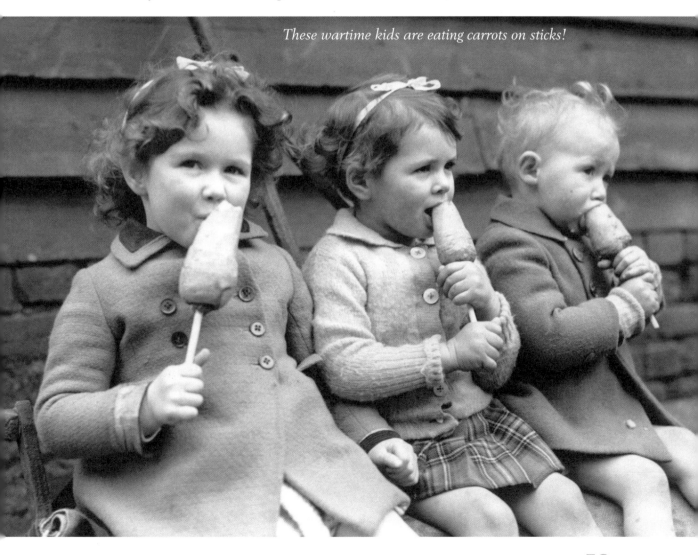

These wartime kids are eating carrots on sticks!

entered the culture of processed, convenience, fast and junk food, which is packed with 'hidden' fats, sugar, salt and a multitude of additives to give bulk, texture, colour and taste (all of which had been 'processed' out). Children now are the offspring of parents who themselves were of the processed food generation, and the 'fresh is best' message has been lost. As already mentioned, children today have foods specifically aimed at them by big business, which are packed with fat, and children's menus in restaurants and, sadly, schools, still reflect this. A school dinner might be a child's major meal of the day, and if that is high in fat (and other undesirables), then overweight if not obesity seems almost inevitable.

Children snack all the time these days as well, something my generation didn't do. I remember a packet of crisps as a luxury once a week or so, a special treat. (I once came across a child with a packed lunch consisting of two packets of crisps, cheesy dippers, a chocolate bar and some boiled sweets!) The trouble with snack-type foods is that they provide such a high proportion of a child's daily energy needs (i.e. calories) that it is hard to find food that is nutrient-rich enough to make up the rest of the daily diet without adding yet more calories. And of course children today take on average very much less exercise than they used to, often staying in to watch television rather than playing football or rugby. (But then, school playing fields are almost a thing of the past as well…)

In 2004, a docu-film called *Super Size Me* followed the fortunes of one Morgan Spurlock, who spent thirty days eating McDonald's meals for breakfast, lunch and dinner. He gained over 7kg in weight, and after twenty-two days Mr Spurlock was also close to a serious liver condition called non-alcoholic steato-hepatitis. His liver had started to absorb fat – in much the same way as a force-fed goose's liver turns to foie gras. He also had a noticeable increase in two types of body fat, the aforementioned cholesterol, as well as triglycerides. (The latter come from refined carbohydrates like burger buns and milkshakes, and they too are known to increase the risk of heart disease and diabetes.)

Such a diet is extreme – and no one (in his or her right mind) would actually eat like that. But if a mere three weeks can bring a grown man's body to near disaster, think what it could do to a much smaller child.

Low-fat diets are very popular these days, as messages about fat and obesity are getting across to people. Children, however, should never be put on any sort of diet, nor made to worry about 'fatness' (there are too many children suffering from food-related diseases like anorexia and bulimia). The larger picture is much the same as that for sugar and salt – that a daily intake of fresh and healthy food will be better than processed foods in which there may be hidden fat, or indeed foods which are obviously fatty, such as hamburgers and chips. But fat, of course, makes certain foods *taste* good to a certain extent, so we can't cut it out altogether. Foods cooked in butter or oil are delicious – just cut down on the amounts. Don't add so much butter to vegetables when serving (if you are serving newly picked carrots, for instance, you won't need any). Spread butter very thinly on bread for sandwiches. Cut visible fat off meats after cooking (the fat moistens and flavours the meat

A school dinner might be a child's major meal of the day…

during cooking). Don't shallow-fry or deep-fry too much – other methods of cooking such as grilling use little or no fat (and fat actually drips off grilled meat). You can't make certain dishes that children love without fat – such as pastry or crumble toppings – but the answer is to cut down on how often you serve them. A home-made meat or fruit pie once a week isn't going to do anyone any harm.

I FEED CHILDREN EVERY DAY, so I know how much they can enjoy their food. I try to provide good honest dishes that will satisfy their hunger and keep them going through the afternoon. I know that what I cook isn't laden with additives, and that it isn't high in other undesirables such as sugar, salt and fat. But what I don't know is what my children eat in the morning before school and at night after school. As I've said before, it's parents who buy and cook food on the whole, and it's at home that most of the healthy eating messages must be established and monitored. Again, it's simply a matter of common sense.

FOOD ALLERGY AND FOOD INTOLERANCE

NONE OF MY OWN CHILDREN REACTED BADLY to foods. They didn't *like* some foods, and therefore couldn't eat them, but they were never sick, or came out in rashes, after eating any particular food. However, since starting work in schools, I have encountered quite a few children who do react badly, and doctors say that allergies and food intolerances in children are on the increase. One of the St Peter's pupils is a case in point. She has potentially life-threatening allergies to eggs, nuts and milk, and although she and her parents are practical and sensible about her problems, they obviously all find it quite difficult. For me, at school, trying to cook something that she can eat each day has proved a challenge, and I have been challenging myself for a few years now. As far as I am concerned, she is a healthy and happy girl, with a good appetite, and it is a pleasure to cook for her.

It is a sad fact that certain foods and drinks can cause adverse reactions in some people. If these reactions recur each time a particular food or drink is taken, this is classified as a food allergy. But true allergies, which can remain throughout life, are quite rare, and most people with food reactions have what are called intolerances, and these can be temporary rather than lifelong. Food allergies and intolerances can trigger conditions such as eczema, asthma, migraine, arthritis, hayfever, digestive problems, coeliac disease, behavioural changes and, the most serious, anaphylactic shock. Lesser symptoms include wind, diarrhoea, catarrh, rhinitis, croup, infant colitis and rashes.

Young babies, whose digestive systems are immature (until about seven months), are very vulnerable to the potential of food allergy or intolerance, particularly if they come from an atopic family, where parents or close relations already suffer from such sensitivities. In the simplest terms, a food might not be properly digested by a baby before being absorbed, and in reaction to foreign proteins in the bloodstream, the body produces antibodies to counter them. These antibodies can become abnormally protective – usually in about one child in five – which means that the next time the body encounters that substance, the antibodies will fight it, thus producing allergic reactions.

To help avoid food allergy and intolerance in children and adults, be careful about what you feed your baby during the first twelve months. The most common allergens are:

Cows' milk Cows' milk is perfect for calves – but not so perfect for small babies. It is not so easily absorbed by babies, as the protein structure is very much more concentrated than that of breast milk (which is protective for the first six months). The same applies to foods made with cows' milk, such as cheese, butter, cream, ice cream and, to a lesser extent, yoghurt. All can lead to allergy. Many children and adults can also become lactose intolerant (unable to digest milk sugars).

Eggs It is often the white of egg that causes problems, so offer only well-cooked yolks at first. Don't cook eggs to a soft stage, as in custards and scrambled eggs, and avoid products containing uncooked egg, such as ice cream, soft meringues and mousses. And, of course, there have been food scares involving eggs.

Wheat Wheat, rye, oats and barley contain gluten, a common allergen. In extreme cases, a child can develop coeliac disease, which affects the intestine's ability to absorb foods, and can lead to malnourishment. Infant rice cereal, which does not contain gluten, is the best cereal to offer at first.

Fish and shellfish These should not be given to a baby until about nine months, because of allergy risk. Try white fish only at first. Shellfish such as mussels can cause anaphylactic shock in vulnerable children and adults. The throat swells in reaction, restricting breathing, and in many cases the outcome can be fatal unless adrenaline is administered.

Nuts and peanuts Being hard, they could cause choking, so have no place in a baby's diet. But even as ground nuts they should be avoided, as these too can cause anaphylactic shock. Children from atopic families should avoid nuts altogether for at least three years.

Citrus fruits and strawberries These can cause contact rashes, because of the acids in the fruit, and also other allergic reactions because of salicylates, naturally occurring chemicals.

Food additives Artificial colourings, flavourings and preservatives should be avoided at all costs, particularly when a child is very small. They are implicated in cases of hyperactivity, lack of concentration, fretfulness, poor co-ordination and insomnia, as well as many allergies. They are contained in a horrifying number of foods and drinks, especially those aimed at children. We all recognize how damaging many of these chemicals can be to *grown* bodies, but think how much more so they are to *growing* bodies.

Revolution

As I was beginning to despair about the food I was being obliged to feed my children at St Peter's, and worry about the future of school dinner ladies in general, the old head, Garth Powell, retired. He was a fantastic head, the old-fashioned sort. (When he left, we all gave him a huge send-off, cooking a complete meal for him and his friends.) The person to be his successor, and my future mentor, was David Maddison (*pictured below left with me*). He's a man with vision who was interested in what my team did in the kitchen, and he soon recognized that we were working extra hours with no extra pay in order to cook as much as we could from scratch and to avoid those packet meals. Serving the best-quality food we could muster was the only way I could see of encouraging the children to stay for dinner – and that had obviously worked, as our numbers had remained stable.

The first thing David did as far as school dinners were concerned was suggest that we might move from Family Service, the one set meal per day. The trouble with Family Service was that if the children didn't like the set meal, they didn't stay. What they called 'Choice' was the alternative, and this meant that we could offer a choice of three to five main courses, and seven to eight puddings. This Choice had always been available to us, but Mr Powell hadn't wanted to change the system. David, however, thought the children might like Choice better, and he suspected that I might too, as I was so obviously bored out of my brain! We still had to serve the same pre-prepared foods, but the children could choose what they liked instead of being faced with just one thing. The numbers immediately went up, which tells its own story.

Around this time, we also got what was called an 'Open Shopping Basket'. Someone in the upper echelons of schools catering had obviously recognized the unease that existed in school kitchens. Within these baskets were flour, sugar, margarine and eggs, etc., so we could begin, although only on a small scale, to cook properly again.

(I wonder if someone had at last realized that CCT didn't work!) Our then client officer, Carol Taylor, after talking to David, got us new mobile trolleys too, which made everything much easier, as we were able to wheel the hot food in the trolleys into the dining hall, giving us a completely new section from which to serve the children. These trolleys brought their own problems though, as we had to have what we called flight trays, airline trays, which we were told were quicker to wash than a plate. Of course they weren't, as they were configured plastic, with lots of indentations in which food could get caught, and were actually miles more difficult to clean properly. But they were *plastic*, which was the whole point as far as they were concerned. They were also multi-coloured, which led to some odd colour combinations: yellow chicken curry in a yellow flight tray is not very pleasant to look at …

The principal trouble with Choice, though, was that the contractors would tell you how many of each chosen dish you could serve. For instance, for a main course, you might want to offer shepherd's pie and fish fingers, but what they would insist on was that 80 per cent of your order had to be fish fingers. Why? Because fish fingers were cheaper. So out of my 200 children, only forty could have shepherd's pie, which isn't a lot. The menu might have looked good – we were serving both meat and fish, after all – but there weren't nearly enough portions, and many children were being disappointed. The same happened with the puddings. We would have the choice to serve yoghurt, fresh fruit salad, cheese and biscuits and a pudding, but we would be obliged to offer 75 per cent pudding, with the other choices much more limited – again because they were more expensive.

In any school cook's contract it says that, within reasonable distances, we can be asked to cover in another school. Any cook in any kitchen could be asked at short notice to travel and, although I had trained up a good team at St Peter's, David became a bit fed up with me always being away. I did too, not liking to be away from the school for too long, and I became almost as frustrated as I had been before. David understood, though, and our relationship continued to grow. We were able to bounce ideas off each other, and I always felt that I was part of the bigger picture, even if I wanted to achieve more than I was able to then. We talked about what had been happening in secondary schools. In 1999, they had had the option to break away from the local authority catering service, and we knew that, in time, primary schools would be able to follow. After one such conversation, he said, 'One day, Jeanette, one day. If you think you can go it alone, I will support you.' Until he said those words, I would never have dreamed I could do such a thing. But this, along with my ladies, is what kept me going.

We had a vision of using nothing but fresh food for our meals, nothing frozen, nothing from a packet.

And my chance finally came in April 2000. The government's new national legislation, which allowed schools three options for running their catering services, was now applied to primaries. They could either continue to use the local authority system (which is what we had been doing), get an external company to provide the whole service for them, or they could run every aspect of the process themselves. As soon as I heard the news, I went straight to David and said, 'How about taking food back in-house?' Quite apart from the cooking, at this point it seemed important to me for the ladies in the kitchen and myself to have guaranteed hours and to feel that we were part of the school as a whole. (My interest in the sourcing of food came much later.)

I knew that I would be taking on a lot more work and a lot more pressure, but I also knew I just had to do it. And luckily David was on my side. Because of our good relationship, he gave me confidence. It was a great sea-change for him, as head teachers don't usually involve themselves too much in school catering (now, years later, he thinks he's Gary Rhodes), but he's one of those people who wants to go that extra mile, and the person you want to go that extra mile for. With his belief in me, I found I was ready to 'go it alone'. We put our initial plans to the school governors and to the parents and we all agreed. They were a community of like-minded people who wanted the best for the children, and we worked very closely together from the start. And continue to do so.

Setting up our own dinner service was a challenge on many levels, but when someone says it can't be done, I dig my teeth in like a terrier and cling on, all the more determined! (My mother will happily confirm that the worst thing anyone can say to me is that I can't possibly do it.) I talked to the ladies in the kitchen about the new plans, for I wanted them to be able to take pride in what they would be doing. The new service would belong to all of us, the whole school, but their input would be essential to the smooth running of the kitchen. So Chris, Alison and Jane Bancroft, the fourth member of the team, talked through every detail over endless cups of tea, from menus to uniforms, from working hours to cleaning days. We had a vision of using nothing but fresh food for our meals, nothing frozen, nothing from a packet, but to do so would take time.

Meanwhile, there was the current budget to contend with, which involved much more mathematics than I had ever encountered before. David and I had to sort out our baseline, to calculate how many children we needed to have staying for lunch in order to pay for the food we would be buying. We eventually worked out that we had to do 115 meals to break even. At this time we were doing an average of 120 meals a day, so we knew that we could make it work. Plus, we had the children who were bringing in packed lunches to convert! We also needed to allow for the wages – mine and the other ladies' in the kitchen – and the running costs. When we had a basic plan, we had to give the county council three months' notice, and I invited our then client officer, Heather Parker, to come in for a chat. She knew what we were trying to achieve, and was not only supportive of our service but also very helpful. I had to know if we could keep our equipment, because if that wasn't possible, we couldn't have done it. However, everything reverted to the school when we opted out – even the new trolleys – which was reassuring (although this is perhaps not universal to every council). We knew that, although the equipment was old, all of us had looked after it well, and it would have to last us at least a year. (Unfortunately Heather left the service so she did not see us complete our first year, but her successor, Liz Dunmore, helped me through every procedure and has become a very good friend. Interestingly, she left the Client Service department to become catering manager of a large secondary school, doing very similar work to us.)

When I stopped to think about it, my potential role as a purchaser of food for 600 meals a week, thirty-eight weeks a year, would give me considerable buying muscle, much, much more than I had ever dreamed possible. It was quite frightening really. In our earlier meetings with the existing catering contractors, it had been made quite clear to us that they didn't think I would be able to get such good deals with suppliers as they could through bulk buying. I was very happy to be able to prove them wrong! For, to my surprise, there was quite a lot of good news. I soon discovered that I would be able to spend more than I had been on the food itself, while keeping the price of a meal in line with every other school in the county. We had been paying about 30–35p for ingredients per child, and

You'd be surprised to see how many potatoes you need to feed 200 hungry mouths.

charging the statutory £1.50 per lunch. Now I could afford 70p a head on ingredients, twice the national average, and still make a profit, because there were no administrators, secretaries or chief executives to pay. In other words, we didn't need to pay for a whole tier of management – my first lesson in big business! It meant hard work for me and our budget was very tight, but being able to spend 50 per cent more than most schools on meals would be worth it. And the prime consideration, notwithstanding the cash question, was that the children would be eating better food.

To begin with, although we had opted out, very little changed. Maybe because I had been working for the authority for so long, I did not know *how* to change. For quite a while we continued serving the same foods, using similar ingredients and some of the same suppliers, but also bringing in more local stuff. This is where my passion for local and organic food was founded.

With everything in place so far as finances, equipment and supply were concerned, we were ready to go. We decided to do it with a bang. For our first lunch – in April 2000 – we opened the school hall to the whole village and prepared lunch for 200 people. What a day! The workload was phenomenal, but we left no detail to chance. You'd be surprised to see how many potatoes you need to feed 200 hungry mouths. As we didn't have the machinery to do it – our 'Rumbler' had been taken away – I went in at five in the morning, stood at the sink and peeled two huge sacks of spuds by hand, which left my hands red raw. And don't get me started on the dishes! I thought we had catered for plenty of people, with a choice of about eight main dishes and six desserts, all for £1.50 – to demonstrate what would be on future menus – but I was wrong. As people started to arrive for our big event, they just didn't seem to stop coming. That's when I said jokingly to David, 'Have you put a sign on the Fosse Way saying "Dinners This Way"?' We'd underestimated the turnout and found ourselves scrambling in the kitchen to get more food on the go. There was a mad panic and cries of 'Jane, more carrots!' and we ended up making lunch for about 300 that day. We were exhausted after making and serving endless portions of all our offerings (see the menu below), but it was a fantastic success. Judging by the numbers, the village must have been empty that lunchtime – even the local press came. That was just the start of our journey.

THE MONTHS JUST FLEW and by the end of the financial year we had made a small profit. Unlike other organizations, it all went back into the kitchen. I was delighted and used the money to buy a new cooker. We needed three in the kitchen now just to cater for the amount of meals we were providing, which had risen from 120 pupils staying for dinner to 180, over 80 per cent of the school. The numbers spoke for themselves.

THE MENU FOR OUR LAUNCH DAY

🍽 *Roast pork, stuffing and gravy*

🍽 *Bacon Pizza. Cheese pizza. Chicken pizza*

🍽 *Chicken tikka jacket potato. Cheese jacket potato.
Tuna mayonnaise jacket potato. Egg and bacon jacket potato*

🍽 *Roast potatoes, broccoli, carrots, coleslaw, stir-fry,
assorted green salad, tomatoes and cucumber*

🍽 *Jelly, ice cream, iced buns, apple crumble,
iced chocolate sponge and custard*

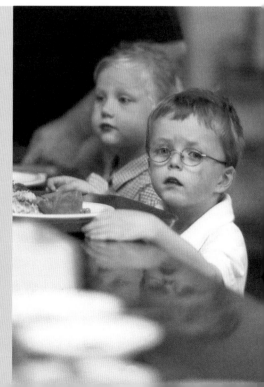

Sourcing Local Ingredients

WHEN WE SET UP the new dinner service at St Peter's, we worked flat out for the first three months, scrubbing, peeling, cooking and cleaning, but although the kids were responding well to our lunches, I didn't think we were making a big enough difference yet to what they were eating. Because I lived in a village and knew many local farmers, we often talked about the pressures they were under to supply good food at cheap prices. These conversations led me to believe that maybe we could make a small difference to our community by sourcing local food. But I still could only afford to use the frozen mince I was supplied and we still made some of the puddings from a packet mix and the custard with dried milk. Some of the ingredients were local, but it was a relatively small proportion of each plate. In a sense we were still in county council mode, and I felt I had to break away from that.

So gradually I started saying to the ladies that we should be serving fresh meat. We sourced some to begin with, but I still wasn't 100 per cent happy, not always knowing its exact origins. This had become desperately important to me – and everyone else in the country – because of the BSE crisis. When I talked to David about wanting to put beef back on the menu (to give the kids variety as well as all of the proteins they need from a balanced diet), I knew it was a controversial idea, as British beef had been banned from school kitchens in Nottinghamshire for about three years. I knew that the only way I could reintroduce it was if we all knew exactly where the meat had come from.

There was only one thing for it. I got into my car and visited local farmers and farm shops to see if anyone might be interested in supplying meat to St Peter's for thirty-eight weeks of the year. Having lived in the area for years, I knew quite a few of the farmers, and I knew what a hard time they had been having. Thirty-eight weeks wasn't fifty-two, but it was a fair proportion of the year, and it would mean a regular income for the farmers. There were conditions, however. The meat would have to be delivered at a certain time (never when the children were in the playground), it could never be delivered late – you can't be left with nothing to feed 200 children! – and it had to come in at a very competitive price. It also had to arrive in child-friendly cuts, small enough for the children to chew and not to provide us with waste. Waste was something we couldn't afford.

> *I got into my car and visited local farmers and farm shops to see if anyone might be interested in supplying meat to St Peter's for thirty-eight weeks of the year.*

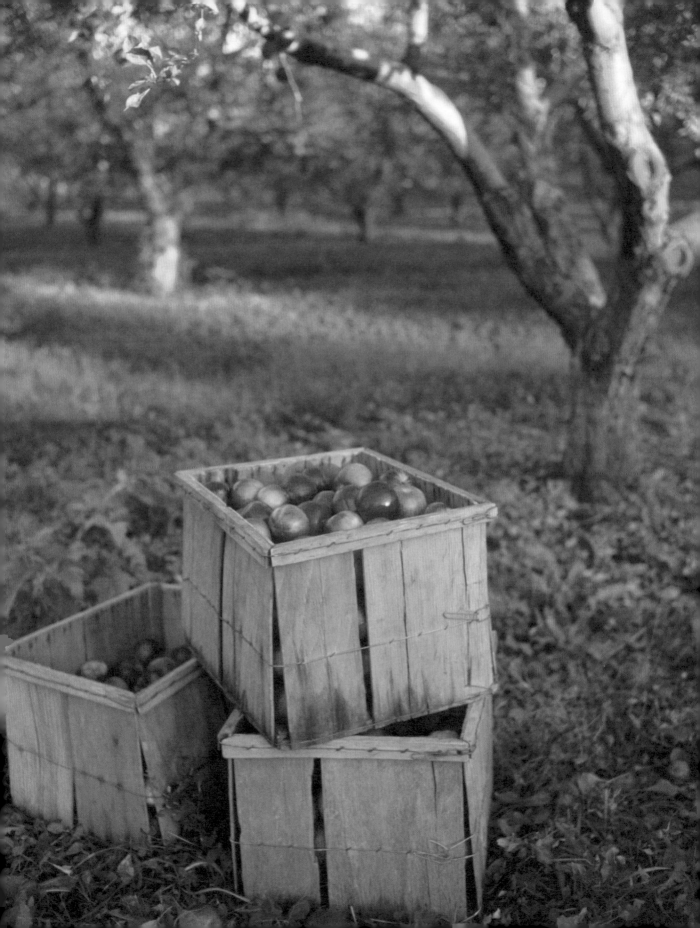

A BRIEF INTRODUCTION TO ORGANICS

GOOD HEALTH AND GOOD FOOD START IN A good soil. If soil is deficient, then so are the plant foods grown in it. These plants don't grow properly, and are prone to disease and pest attacks. Conventional intensive agriculture combats this with the use of pesticides to kill disease, weeds and pests, and artificial chemical fertilizers to promote growth. The result is plant foods that are full of harmful residues. (Recent research has shown that pesticide residues, sometimes as high as six times the recommended safety level, can be found in intensively farmed food.) These residues can be ingested by animals that feed on them, and by humans who eat both the plants and animals. The soil itself is depleted, as well as retaining those same harmful residues, which in turn means more chemical fertilization is needed. Side effects of this type of farming are the disappearance of a growing number of animals, birds and insects, many of which actually benefit soil and growing plants, and millions of pounds spent annually on removing toxic chemicals from rivers and streams. Food-related diseases and food scares are becoming increasingly common, and more and more connections are being made between these and intensive agriculture.

Organic farming aims to counter all these conventional intensive farming practices, and the health of the soil is paramount to the whole operation. This involves maximizing nutrients in the soil by utilizing plant and animal waste as manure and compost, and by rotating crops and livestock to control weeds, pests and diseases. No pesticides or fertilizers are used (although an approved range of mostly plant-based treatments can be permitted). Food animals are also reared without the routine use of the drugs, antibiotics, growth promoters and wormers commonly found in most conventional livestock farming. Animals are also free range, with access to the outdoors, and with comfortable housing. By working with Nature rather than against it, the organic way of farming produces plants and animals that, because they are inherently healthy, are naturally disease-resistant, requiring no other assistance from the producer.

Organic food costs more to produce than non-organic. Crop yields are often lower because organic farms do not use quick-fix solutions (fertilizers, etc.). Manual weeding (instead of herbicides) will probably add to the farmers' costs. Organic livestock will take longer to reach a marketable size, lacking the growth promoters and feedstuffs of intensive farming. And, of course, organic farms are still in the minority, so their produce is always likely to be more expensive than that bought and sold cheaply by the supermarkets. The bottom line is that the food we buy is actually too cheap, something we've got far too used to. Think about what a bean from Kenya really costs in terms of air miles and so on. And of course many organic products have to be imported anyway. If budget is limited, my first preference would be for organic vegetables and fruit – the fresh things – followed closely by organic meat. If the meat is more expensive, choose it carefully, perhaps buying a joint that will stretch beyond one roast meal, or cheaper cuts of the animal that will stew well. I'd rather have a really good piece of meat once a week than inferior meat every day. The organic store-cupboard foods you can buy now are good, but not so essential, I feel, as the fresher foods.

In the UK, organic farmers and producers have to work to a set of standards, which are monitored by a number of certification bodies, chief among them the Soil Association (see page 107).

My trail eventually led me to a local farm shop at Hockerton. After I had talked to them at length, they became very supportive of what I was trying to do, and were keen to help when they realized that they would have a regular and major order – with a regular income – and that their meat would be eaten by local schoolchildren. The owner took me to their suppliers so that I could see the free-range farms where their meat came from. I'd been looking for quality, delivery, cost and continuity and I had finally found it. I came to know everything about the meat and the animals, from what they were fed to the fact that they were slaughtered about fifteen minutes' drive away from the farm (which meant little stress for the animals – something that has been ruined since the introduction of new EC abattoir regulations). David teased that I probably knew all of the cows' names too!

Once I had found my new meat supplier, I was happy with the produce and so were the children. We then had not only beef, but a range of local chicken, turkey, pork, ham, bacon and lamb to put on our menu. Some of the meat was from rare breeds, such as Gloucester Old Spot pigs and Dexter cows, some was organic as well, and my ladies in the kitchen all noticed the difference in quality, both in the cooking and in the taste. Especially Jane who, when asked what she liked about the new system, said, 'Because I like to eat the food now.' And she does, she always makes sure she has her dinner! I now buy my meat from Gonalston Farm shop (*opposite*), owned by Georgina and Ross Mason.

The next thing was the milk. We had been using dried milk, as fresh milk was very expensive. I used to occasionally buy milk from the local post office cum village shop in East Bridgford, which was run by Charles and Jennifer Holt, both very big in organic food. I must confess that I used to spend hours talking to Charles, who was – and is – very knowledgeable and informative. The more I listened, the more sense the concept of organics made, although I knew I wouldn't be able to buy organic for some time. In the end it was I who sourced the local milk, through the farm shop where I got my meat. A relative of someone at the shop was a dairy farmer, and as they were just up the road, I

The majority of suppliers I had been using were offering jet-lagged vegetables that had been stored for months and had probably travelled for miles.

went to see them. Once again, price and delivery were the prime considerations, but Newfield Dairy was happy to fall in with my plans. And, of course, I was pleased because they were local, and also because I could follow the same 'audit trail' as I had with the beef and other meats: I saw how the cows were kept, how they were milked, saw that the dairy was clean – for you can't be too careful when you are catering for a high-risk group like young children.

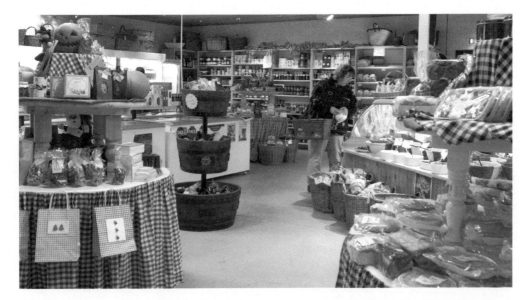

(The farmers, Ann and John Pogson, have a daughter, Carmen, who has plans to revive a forgotten local cheese, which, if it happens, might very well turn up on the St Peter's menu.)

Ironically, Charles is now using the same dairy for his milk at the post office. And the children were quick to respond to my use of fresh milk, for we could now make *real* custard, virtually an impossibility with dried milk. 'Ooh, Mrs Orrey, this is so creamy!' was the response, and some of the children now actually eat bowls of custard by itself. Having for years made up pints of watery milk using powder, I was happy too, as that full-cream milk was exactly what the children should be having for their growing bones and teeth.

Then I asked myself, why stop at buying locally produced meat and milk? Why couldn't we purchase potatoes and vegetables in the same way, preferably local and organic? Because Jeanette, I remember answering myself, you don't have a Rumbler! Never mind, I thought, I will peel the potatoes by hand, one sack will feed all of the children and maybe they will notice the difference. I was no scientist but I knew the ones supplied in whitening could never be as good as fresh, and who knows what was in those chemicals (and there had been so many food scares, from salmonella and CJD, to antibiotics in chicken and dioxins in milk). The majority of suppliers I had been using were offering jet-lagged vegetables that had been stored for months and had probably travelled for miles, which seemed stupid when we lived in the middle of a huge agricultural area – Nottinghamshire itself, and with Lincolnshire and Leicestershire so close. So I phoned an organic shop not too far away who said they could provide me with fresh produce. Great, I thought, but they proved to be too expensive and not that reliable. So I got back into my car and started another search.

Some time later, I took a trip out to the organic Haywood Oaks Farm in Blidworth to see if they could supply us with plenty of fresh vegetables on a regular basis. The owner, Richard Thomas, agreed. He and his farm manager, Jamie Speed-Andrews, admitted that they had not done anything on this scale before, but they were willing to give it a go – and they were happy to accept all my conditions on delivery and price. They were also very happy that I was prepared to accept what the supermarkets define as 'outgrades' – vegetables that might be less than perfect in shape and size, and which, horrifyingly, were often used as cattle feed or, worse, landfill. The Haywood Oaks response was exactly what I wanted to hear. It's all very seasonal, of course, but I like that – and I certainly like how appreciative the children are when we serve them the first of the new carrots, for instance. They go mad, as these newly dug carrots are so packed with sweetness. We buy courgettes, parsnips, leeks, broccoli and numerous other vegetables as well, when in season, and we get the kids to try everything. I now also have a local producer, Maxey's, who grow their own vegetables.

I still use some frozen food, and some foods from cans. I have to, as I need a back-up just in case someone's crop goes wrong, for instance. Frozen peas are good in any case, famously frozen almost as soon as they are picked and podded. Frozen sweetcorn is processed (although that is not a good word to use in this context) in the same way, frozen as soon as picked from the plant – and the children love its sweetness and colour. I buy organic seasonal fruit and salad as well, but quite a lot of the time I have to rely on imported, as much of the fruit the children like is not grown in this country. We can't source local oranges, for instance, and often we can't even get local and home-grown apples, as almost all our orchards, locally and nationally, have been grubbed up. You've got to be realistic, as nothing can be perfect. It's not a perfect world.

I can afford the luxury of frozen food, as with some of that first year's profits, we bought a freezer – and, even more luxurious, a Rumbler! We couldn't afford new, so I ended up calling round the catering 'graveyards' to find second-hand machinery. We made sure it was all in good working order so that we didn't get any nasty surprises. All of us in the kitchen marvelled at putting the first sack of potatoes through our reconditioned Rumbler and seeing them come out clean and white in minutes. The machine paid for itself in about three months, and what a difference it has made to our lives. Those machines, especially the freezer, have also helped me save money. With the meat, for instance, I could now order in for two weeks instead of one, so I could have one week of fresh, and freeze the meat for the second week. By doing so, not only was I getting the meat at a better rate, but I was also saving on delivery, as they didn't charge for that on a fortnightly basis. Everything was starting to come together.

WHERE TO BUY ORGANIC FOOD

ORGANIC FOOD IS NOW AVAILABLE THROUGH A large range of outlets. Box schemes are important in this; often you know intimately the local farm where the foods included in the box were grown, something that is very close to my heart. These boxes can be delivered to an individual household or to a central drop-off point. The vegetables and fruit will be fresh, but they may be a little dirty (we have become so used to the pristine look of pre-washed supermarket veg). They may not last very long either, one of the main criticisms of organic food – but why try to keep something that is so fresh? And sometimes the only reason that non-organic foods last on the shelves is because they have been treated with preservatives: I know which I'd prefer. Home delivery is another scheme, whereby plant foods as well as groceries (such as dairy products, bread or meat), often chosen from a catalogue or, nowadays, a website, are brought to the customer.

Organic farm shops, farm gate stalls and market stalls are available to those living in the country. In towns and cities, farmer's markets supply foods that were grown within a certain distance from the marketplace (in London, within 100 miles of the M25), but the stallholders are not all necessarily organic. At outlets like these, you might find the unusual vegetable or fruit that you wouldn't find elsewhere, for organic producers do not have to stick to the monoculture demanded by large food companies and supermarkets.

Many independent retailers in towns and cities are now dedicated to organic produce. And most of the large supermarkets are now offering a limited range of organic foods. Because of the nature of their business, though, there are seasonal variations in availability, and much of their produce can be imported from abroad.

The Soil Association can help with accessing local organic outlets (see page 280).

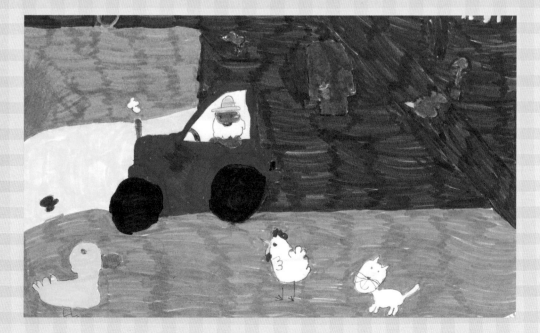

And What About the Children?

R EINTRODUCING WHAT I CALL 'proper' food into the school was not an instant operation, simply because you cannot change the menu overnight and expect the children to like and eat it straight away. These kids were used at school to eating chicken nuggets, burgers and chips loaded with additives, E-numbers and salt to make them more palatable. Encouraging children to change their eating habits is not an easy task, but there are a few strategies, some of which I outline below. There is no quick fix, but it's worth persevering.

I remember cooking my first totally organic roast dinner in the school kitchen. I was so proud to be serving it, and devastated when the lunch trays were returned almost untouched. Most of the organic chicken went straight into the bin, and I went home crying because the children didn't like it. At the time, I couldn't for the life of me understand why, but now I think it is because children these days aren't used to chewing. They've grown used to the soft texture of those overprocessed sausages, burgers and chicken nuggets, which can simply be swilled around in the mouth and

They've grown used to the soft texture of those overprocessed sausages, burgers and chicken nuggets, which can simply be swilled around in the mouth and then swallowed.

then swallowed. They have forgotten how to chew real food – a disaster for their mouth and jaw formation (see pages 84–5) – and it must also have tasted strange at first, without that kick of salt and sugar. So, the next time, we cut the meat into smaller pieces and told them that this was 'real food', asking, 'Do you like it?', and telling them, 'See what you think'. This was key. I realized that I had to talk to the children about their likes and dislikes, and their parents too. So part of my strategy now is to go round the dining hall at lunchtime and sit with the children for a few minutes at each table, talking to them, asking how they are, whether they like the food, whether there is anything they would like to see on the menu which we have not got on. I also talk to David, the teaching staff and the midday supervisors, asking for their opinions on the menu, and whether they think the children are happy with their school meals. We also have a school council and a catering committee, both of which hold regular meetings. In essence we try to include the children every step of the way to ensure that it is *their* meal service.

I adopted a different strategy with another favourite at St Peter's, chicken nuggets. I read a newspaper article to the kids of Year 6 (11–12-year-olds), which described in gory detail what the nuggets contained. According to Felicity Lawrence, chicken nuggets are often made from MRM (mechanically recovered meat, which includes skin and other less savoury parts), then this slurry is bound together with polyphosphates and emulsifying gums, and additives, salts and sugars are added (to make them taste of anything at all). Then, of course, the nuggets are floured, battered, breadcrumbed and deep-fried. One packet of nuggets tested by a county council trading standards department contained only 16 per cent meat, 30 per cent less than claimed – but 46 per cent is a fairly low proportion of meat anyway. After that enlightenment, not one child in my school would eat processed chicken nuggets any more – and anyway, home-made are so much better (see page 131).

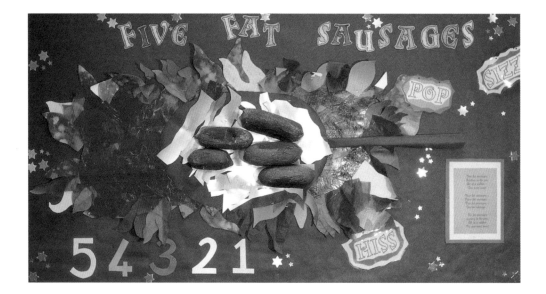

I soon realized too that the kids were vulnerable to peer pressure and that there was nothing more powerful, even when it came to food. So we asked them to try new dishes and to give us their honest opinion. We found that there would generally be a consensus: if one didn't like it, twenty others wouldn't either. We started to talk to the children about why they didn't like a dish, what they thought would improve it, and what would make it nice. And if the majority didn't want to eat it, we promised not to serve the same thing again. And we didn't, because you have to stick to your word with children or they won't trust you. Peer pressure worked in a different way when we were trying to find a local

Kids were vulnerable to peer pressure and there was nothing more powerful, even when it came to food.

sausage that the children would like. We got together a little tasting panel of eight Year 6 children to taste some eight to nine sausages. When they had chosen the one they liked best, and they all agreed, we cooked it for school lunch one day. I arranged it so that the tasting panel came in first in the queue. They chose the sausages, then went and sat down at a special table. Almost without exception, the rest of the queue wanted those sausages, and I'm afraid we didn't have quite enough. Never, ever underestimate peer pressure!

Another reason for keeping faith with the children was because buying locally was proving to be expensive and sticking to the budget was tough. What went into the bin became almost as important to us as what went into the children's mouths! So I regularly asked the kids what they thought as I sat with them at their tables at the end of lunch break. I also spoke to the staff and invited the parents to the school. Even at this stage, and in school, eating together as a family and showing your children that you enjoy good food yourselves is important. I worked more hours than I care to think about, but I never gave up on the belief that it was the right thing to do.

Knowing that we couldn't introduce a completely healthy but alien menu overnight, we decided to make the transformation a gradual process. We served the kind of food that the kids had been used to for four days of the week and replaced that with a good-quality, healthy meal on the fifth. This was usually a Wednesday, when I would do a roast – and I could see that it was working, because the numbers always went up on that day (and they still do!). Even at that stage it was a big improvement, as all of the ingredients were fresh and local, organic if possible. If we served fish fingers and chicken burgers they would be the best quality we could afford and without additives. Little by little we took away the processed foods, and brought in the fresh. We slowly increased the salads and vegetables, and used lean meats in traditional recipes, made in the way the children said they preferred. (I'm afraid they are not keen on anything currently fashionable such as pink lamb; it has to be quite well cooked, even now.) It was all about re-educating children about food, giving them the opportunity to explore new tastes and textures, and letting them make decisions. By asking the parents to come into school, to look at what the children were learning and what they were eating, I think we were re-educating them as well. For if what we had started in St Peter's were properly to succeed, the message had to be carried over into the home environment. It's a joint initiative, and parents and schools (and dinner ladies) have to work together.

At St Peter's we now serve a five-day menu of home-made, fresh, local and sometimes organic dinners, with lots of choice and variety. And the kids tell me what

Little by little we took away the processed foods, and brought in the fresh.

they think. Molly, aged eleven, says that my 'shepherd's pie, broccoli and carrots is tops' while Anna, also aged eleven, says that her favourite is 'the home-made macaroni cheese' which I serve with salad or vegetables. But we're not killjoys, so occasionally we give our kids chicken burgers, chips and beans followed by iced buns, and they love it. The difference is that the chicken burgers are good quality, made from chicken breast, the chips are home-made, and the beans have reduced levels of salt and sugar. Because they are only eating this kind of food once in a while, they are still being provided with a nutritious and balanced diet.

I have had letters from parents thanking me for improving their kids' diets and comments from teachers who say that the children concentrate far better in the afternoons with a good meal inside them. Kids need sustenance to get them through the day, let alone when they are out on the playing field. I love it when parents bring their children to school at 8.45 a.m., about the time that I could be making cookies or sponges, and I hear them in the hallways saying, 'Mmmm, what's that delicious smell?'

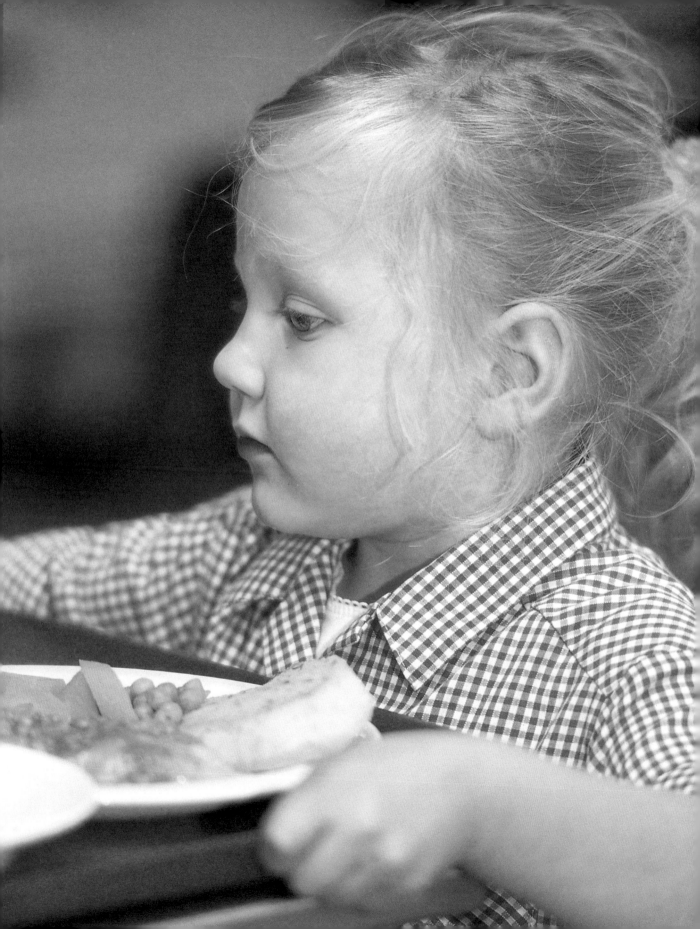

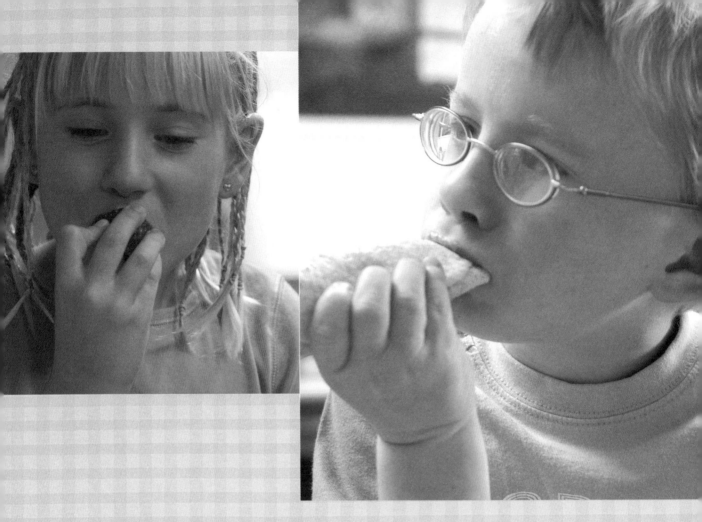

CHEWING IS GOOD

IN THE 1930S, AN AMERICAN DENTIST studied and recorded the jaw and mouth formation of several isolated ethnic groups around the world – Eskimos (Inuits), Polynesians, Australian Aborigines, among others. They all lived on varied and natural diets, and many of their foods had to be chewed well (as all foods should be). The combination of good diet and good chewing meant that both children and adults had wide and well-formed jaws, allowing well-spaced teeth, with little tooth decay. Only a generation later, by which time these peoples had been exposed to westernized processed foods such as

white flours and sugars – not so natural, and not so much chewing involved – he found that the children had less well-formed jaws and dental arches, and that many of them were suffering from tooth decay because their teeth were overcrowded. Dr Weston Price's book, *Nutrition and Physical Degeneration*, was illustrated by graphic before and after photographs.

If this deterioration could occur so quickly, within one generation, I hate to think what might be happening to the mouths of our children today, who have been, and still are, so exposed to highly processed foods. Many of today's foods

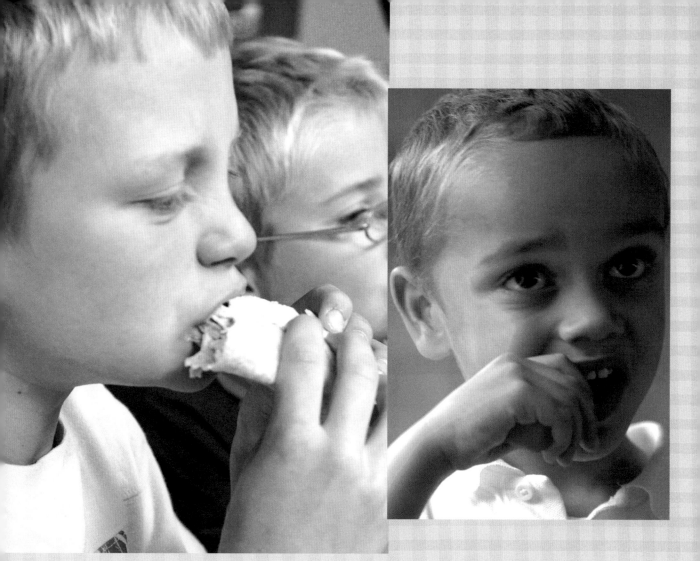

are so refined that they hardly require any chewing at all. I well remember my heartbreak of a few years ago when my carefully cooked organic chicken was left uneaten on the plates (see page 79). The children, used to the softness of foods like chicken nuggets, could not cope with the tougher texture of that chicken.

Chewing is an art that must be learned, and it is vital for jaw and mouth health. Lessons can start as early as a baby's first year. Once a baby has gone beyond the first puréed food stage, he should be introduced to foods with a rougher texture – even before the first

teeth appear (confirmed by one of the findings of ALSPAC, see page 19). The act of chewing stimulates the flow of blood to the jaw, which helps in the growth and formation of the jaw. This in turn allows more room for teeth – and the more room there is for teeth, the less decay there will be, as food will not so easily get caught.

When the first little teeth appear, chewing can still be useful: something crunchy, like an apple or some toast, can help keep both gums and teeth in good condition. And the same goes for second teeth, in both children and adults.

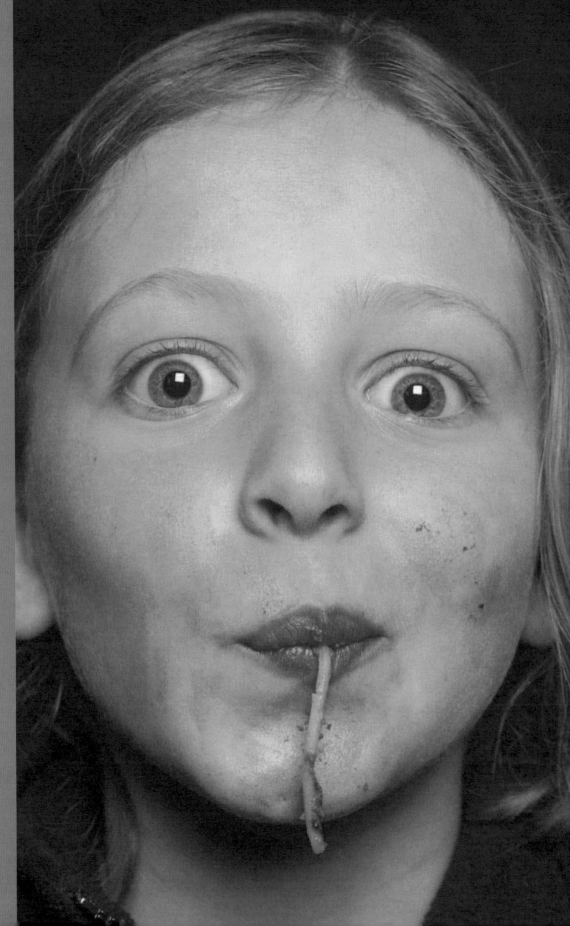

I T WAS ALL HAPPENING as the end of our first independent year approached. Before long, David, the headmaster, who knew me all too well, asked me what my next move was. I told him that I wanted to ask Charles and Jennifer, the owners of the local post office, if they would like us to supply them with fresh filled rolls to sell at lunchtime. It was the only shop in the village, along with the newsagents, and I saw an opportunity to make some extra money to plough back into our dinner service as well as to become part of the wider community. We started off small, and soon started to make about a hundred fresh rolls a week, as they have proved to be very popular.

The dinner take-up numbers remained fairly constant, except on Wednesdays, which was 'roast' day (everyone's favourite), when the percentage went up to 85 per cent and often even higher. The numbers were also boosted by several newcomers. The more I had got involved in the school and with the school curriculum, the more I could see opportunities in which I could get even *more* involved. (Food is a great leveller, after all.) The school curriculum for Year 6 was covering citizenship, and David and I thought, rather than just teach them about the importance of community, why not actually introduce the children to a major part of their own community – the older folk – so that they could get to know each other. And so we formulated the idea of the Wednesday Senior Citizens' Luncheon Club. Several old people from the village come in and eat with Year 6, and I can't tell you how heart-warming it is seeing those kids listening to snippets of living history, local and national, and all of them laughing and enjoying eating together. One lady, then about eighty-five, got to eat with her grandson once a week, and she had us in stitches once remembering how, as a former pupil of the school, she used to have to scrub the floors! We also decided that parents could come in for school dinner if they liked – quite important when the babies come in for the first time – and we have had a very good take-up on that as well. On any given day during the week, we might have four to five mothers (with the occasional father), perching on the tiny chairs at the low tables, tucking in, and not looking at all uncomfortable! (For this, we charge adults £2.00.)

Since that first great day at St Peter's when we served lunch for 300, we had come a long way. I could now be confident that more children in the school were getting a good meal in the middle of the day. As we were using produce from known local sources, this meant that a close watch would be kept on quality and any problems could be dealt with quickly and easily. We still weren't 100 per cent local, but I aimed to do more – as well as include more organic produce. But I knew that, from my increasing knowledge of the principles of the organic movement, that the use of local produce had many benefits, not least for my own particular schoolchildren. Primarily it involved fewer 'food miles' (the distances travelled in producing and distributing food). Fewer food miles in turn meant fewer emissions from delivery lorries and less traffic congestion, less distress to animals because they were less likely to be transported long distances, and less packaging and fewer chemicals needed to preserve food for longer periods. We incorporated some of these 'green' ideas into the curriculum as well, to boost the children's environmental, health and animal-welfare awareness and knowledge. With all this, I felt we were educating them and their families about many aspects of food perhaps unconsidered before, as well as encouraging local farmers who were using sustainable agricultural methods.

We were also helping to support the local economy in ways I didn't understand at first. I could appreciate that if my money for milk was going to Newfield Dairy instead of to the central county council contractor, that money was being spent and accrued locally. But it wasn't until a few years later that I discovered just how valuable that local sourcing could be. An economic concept called LM3, which stands for Local Multiplier 3, has calculated that every pound spent in the local economy is actually worth very much more than that initial pound. For instance, if I give my money to the farmers, then the farmers spend *their* money (on giving local people employment, say), and the people employed by me *and* by the farmers spend *their* money in the area, everything is being generated and spent within the local community, thus benefiting the local economy. My meat bill last year, for instance, was about £5,300, but to the local economy it was worth about £13,800. Similarly with my milk bill of £600; in the local economy it is worth about £1,690. (If we bought from an outside supplier, a large food conglomerate, for instance, my money would go out of the area, perhaps even abroad, and certainly probably to shareholders.) The beneficial mathematics of this seems amazing to me, and we are only one school. Imagine if fifty or all the schools in Nottinghamshire were to do this. And think about how we could *all* do this in our own communities.

We also made a few other changes to the way we served food to the children. I truly believe that you eat more, and eat more contentedly, if you are in a happy-looking place. So we got some blue gingham, wipeable tablecloths, which immediately transformed the school hall into a dining hall. We got rid of the plastic flight trays, and bought plain white china plates, as well as some proper cutlery. This might have seemed extravagant, but to us it made sense, and I think the children appreciate it. I've been in quite a few primary schools in the last few years, and more and more of them are taking on board what we have done and achieved at St Peter's. Kitchen staff and teachers tell me that the children are far calmer, with fewer arguments and incidents than previously.

Changes in the Curriculum

FOOD ITSELF ALSO BECAME part of the curriculum at St Peter's, and it is one of the things I feel most proud about. I passionately believe that children who know about the principles of food – if these are taught in an easy and fun way, and taught early (they're never to young to learn) – will know about eating well, will cook and eat well in the future, and will pass on their knowledge to the next generation. Good food in the middle of the day is only part of the story, though: food in the curriculum can also involve every other school subject – maths, history, geography, art, science and English. We have developed projects for each year, and these have been very popular, not only with the children. With what we call our 'whole school approach', the ladies in the kitchen feel as if they belong, and that their opinions are valued. The children respond because what is taught in the classroom is also carried out in the dining hall.

Year 1 (five-year-olds)

So that they can see where I am buying their food, we take them to one of the organic arable farms that supply our school kitchen. They see how potatoes, carrots, parsnips and courgettes are grown. Gemma Baines, their teacher, and I go with them, and they all meet the person I deal with, Jamie Speed-Andrews, the farm manager. Richard Thomas, who owns the farm, has been very supportive of this idea of reconnecting children with their food – although some children, I must admit, were more interested in the rabbit burrows (but you have to plant the seeds).

We wanted them to learn where their food *goes* to as well, so we took them to one of our local supermarkets (Waitrose). The staff were very good with the children, taking them around the organic section, showing them where the deliveries came in and telling them where the lorries were coming from and from how far away. They also set quizzes for the children.

These five-year-olds also make a fruit salad, but one with a purpose. They meet and talk to the senior citizens who come for lunch on Wednesdays, and ask them what fruit they like. They have a simple chart on which they make drawings of different fruit (art) then two columns of likes and don't likes (English), which they have to add up (maths). The following week they make the fruit salad, again writing down what they will need (e.g. chopping board, knife, dish, apron, as well as the fruit itself), and at lunchtime they give it to their senior citizen partner.

These young children have become very food aware, something I am very proud of. Because of the many press, TV and other media visits to the school, they have also become very media savvy now, as a conversation between two five-year-olds showed.

One asked, 'Is it Sky TV today?' 'No,' said the other, 'that was yesterday, silly. This is the BBC!' Oh well …

Year 2 (six- to seven-year-olds)

These children designed a healthy plate. Their teacher, Kate Watson, had spent weeks talking to them about food, and I went into the classroom as well to explain about protein, fat and carbohydrate, and the importance of fruit and vegetables, pitching it at a level they could grasp. I also took in a large trolley piled high with different foods, explaining why some were good for you and others should be an occasional treat. They then made a 'healthy plate' like a collage. Pictures of different foods were cut out of magazines and stuck on paper plates. These then made a display for their classroom. So I suppose you could say that was a combination of botany, nutrition and art!

Year 3 (seven- to eight-year-olds)

Judy O'Leary, their teacher (and also the deputy head), set them the task of designing a menu for a party. What an eye opener that was! Some did a teddy bears' picnic, some did a football tea, and one young lady devised a menu for a party by the swimming pool, complete with champagne flutes (she will go far). They also designed menu cards, some tied with ribbon, so you had to open them to see what was on offer. These were made into a display, complete with the champagne glasses.

Year 4 (eight- to nine-year-olds)

The children taught by Sue Cains had to design a healthy yoghurt, using natural yoghurt as a base. The first year they did this, the 'filling' was chocolate drops and flakes, hundreds and thousands, marshmallows, Smarties, fruit pastilles, etc. I had to judge the competition, which was no joke as there were thirty-two children in the class and I had to taste every single yoghurt! Anyway, this last year they did the same again, but when I went into the classroom, it smelt like a fruit factory. Every fruit possible was there, and the children were at pains to tell me it was either local or organic. What a difference a year had made. They had understood the thinking behind what we are trying to achieve, and by taking it into the classroom and reinforcing the message in the dining hall, it had been taken thoroughly on board.

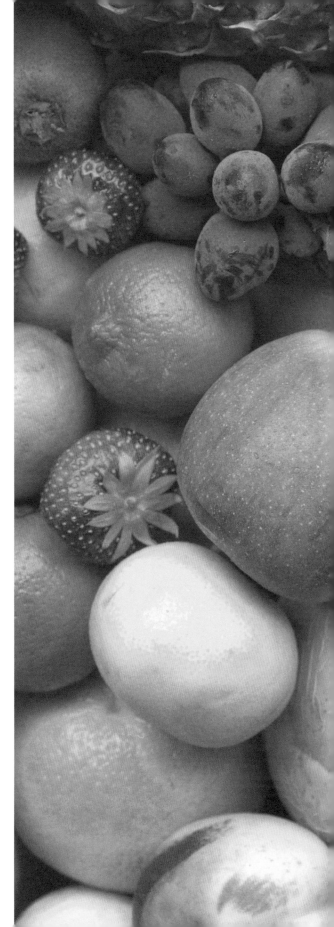

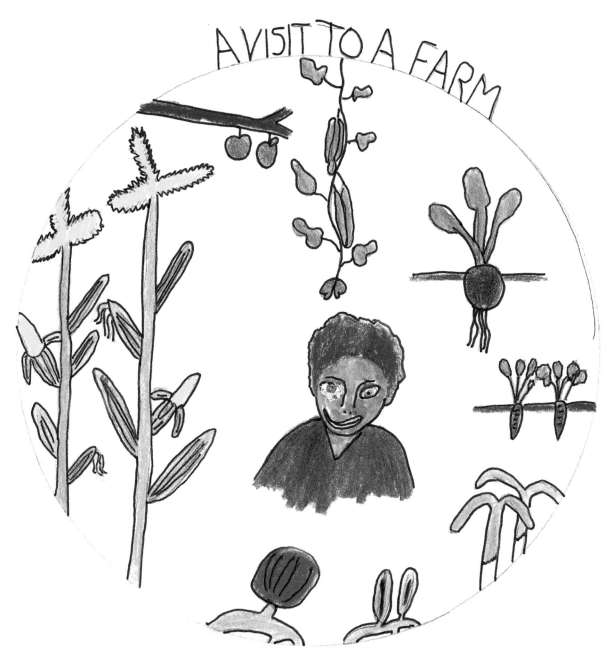

A VISIT TO A FARM

Year 5 (nine- to ten-year-olds)

Their project was to design a healthy menu. Their teacher, Joe Archer, asked me to talk to them about what was healthy and what was not, something to be done quite carefully as I don't want to scare children into being frightened of food (there are enough eating disorders out there already). So I gave a talk that was the wrong way round, if you like. I started by asking the children what they thought was bad for them. The answers came thick and fast – chocolate, chips, burgers, etc. When I asked them why they thought these were bad for them, they come back with: they make you fat, they give you spots, they're unhealthy. Then I was able to ask them if it would be better if you had them only occasionally. I don't want to say to children, no, you can't have that. If you ban foods, that only makes them more attractive. I believe that nothing is really bad for you so long as it is taken in moderation.

So off they went to design their menus. Joe and I judged the entries, and two boys won. Ryan Day gave us:

- *Home-made beefburger*
- *Fresh mixed vegetables*
- *Jacket wedges*
- *Apple pie and custard*

Tom Crossland was the other winner with:

- *Sweet and sour chicken in a tortilla wrap*
- *Stir-fry vegetables*
- *Fresh fruit salad*

Both were very simple menus, but with good wholesome food. I bought the boys a book token each and then suggested we cook and serve the winning menus to the whole school, with Tom and Ryan helping. I bought them chefs' hats and aprons, and nearly the whole school stayed for dinner that day. I got it wrong, though. I always have to judge what is going to be the first to go, and I decided on the beefburger. How wrong can you get, as the sweet and sour chicken went like lightning. Oh well, that taught me a lesson: never underestimate children.

Year 6 (ten- to eleven-year-olds)

Their teacher, Marg Finch, set them the task of designing, packaging and selling a healthy snack bar. She invited me to talk to the children about the kinds of things they would put into the bar. I mentioned that some other children might have allergies to nuts, or to dairy foods such as butter, so they really had to think about what they would put into the bar. If they put fresh fruit in, would it keep? Designing the wrapping was an extra art lesson, and when a teacher from our local secondary school also came to speak to them about marketing, and how to maximize the potential of their product, they were being taught lessons about many things not normally in the school curriculum. Food *can* be fun!

Children in the Kitchen

THE KITCHEN IS ACTUALLY rather a dangerous place for young children, but as it is a room where families spend quite a lot of time, it ought to be made as safe as possible.

|●| Keep all dangerous substances in a high cupboard, not under the sink – unless you have childproof locks. Only keep unbreakable things like pots and pans in drawers or cupboards your child can reach.

|●| Check the heat of your oven door when it is at full blast. Quite a few oven doors get very hot indeed, and a small child could be burned if he touches the door.

|●| Avoid deep-frying. This is the most potentially dangerous of all cooking methods, and thousands of accidents, often involving children, happen every year. A moment's distraction, answering the phone perhaps, and a chip pan could catch light.

|●| Use the back burners on the stove top if you have small children about, and get into the habit of turning saucepan handles towards the back of the cooker rather than the front.

|●| Make sure that there are no loose wires or dangling flexes a child could pull or trip over – or you yourself!

But the kitchen is also a place where children can have fun, whether cooking, growing things, participating or just watching. Even the smallest child can learn through 'cooking', and allowing them to 'help' you will stimulate them, and make them more interested in the end result.

|●| One of the things my boys liked best when they were little was 'printing'. Cut root vegetables into chunks and carve out a pattern or decoration on one of the sides. This side can then be dipped into ink or paint (protect your table top and floor well!) and printed on to paper.

|●| Let them grow something for themselves. The easiest thing is mustard and cress: you simply scatter the seeds on a damp base (blotting paper or kitchen paper) in a container (a plastic box from the supermarket or an old egg box), and leave for about a week, sprinkling with water daily.

|●| You could get them to grow beansprouts. Put a couple of tablespoons of dried beans (not red kidney), peas or lentils into an empty jam jar, rinse with water, and put a piece of J-cloth over the top, securing with an elastic band. Store in a warm, dark place and rinse the beans daily. After about five days, the beans will have germinated and sprouted. (A major advantage of this is that the sprouts are very nutritious – much more so than the original bean. Use them within a couple of days, in salads, salad sandwiches and stir-fries.)

|●| Avocado stones can be set over water until they shoot, but this might be too lengthy a process for smaller children. They might enjoy putting parsnip or pineapple tops in a saucer with water, and seeing them develop roots and shoots. Even sweet pepper seeds and orange pips can germinate in earth, and develop into a miniature plant, if kept in a warm enough place.

|●| If you have a garden, children can grow some vegetables by themselves (with supervision). Radishes are easy, and

they grow fast as well, an advantage with impatient learner gardeners. Let them help you harvest your vegetables and fruit – they would like digging for potatoes, and their keen eyes would soon spot a hidden bean, pea pod or gooseberry. William, my middle son, was always in the garden with his dad, and his sharp eyes helped keep the snail and slug population down (he kept them in a bucket).

🍽 Pastry is popular as a sort of edible play-dough. When you're using pastry (home-made or bought), give a child a few pieces to shape, roll, decorate and flavour (within limits). You can buy small rolling pins – or use a piece of dowelling. Biscuit cutters are useful. Or children can help you by making pie decorations – leaves, balls, apple shapes or tassels.

🍽 They can help make things like mince pies: rolling the pastry, putting the mincemeat in, adding the top. They could wrap pastry around some fruit (a piece of apple or pear, a stoned plum or apricot, or some berries), for an instant fruit tart.

🍽 A stiff pastry-like mixture can be made from flour, salt and water, with a little oil. This can be rolled, shaped, then baked, when it hardens well. The shapes can then be painted and glazed (use clear nail varnish). Children could make presents, ornaments and Christmas decorations (remember to leave a hole for the string).

🍽 Home-made biscuits are great fun for everyone to make. Children could help prepare and mix the dough, roll it out, cut into shapes and decorate.

Gingerbread men would also be popular, and the chocolate krispies on page 265 are good for children to make too.

🍽 Let even the smallest child help in food preparation in some safe way. If you make them feel they can do it, they will acquire confidence and probably do it rather well. You could, for instance, let smaller children sieve some flour and sugar into a bowl for a cake, then help you mix in the liquid. Older children could chop, grate or slice – or indeed prepare one whole element of a meal, from washing or peeling a vegetable, say, through to cooking it, or grilling a chop.

🍽 Get them to top their own pizzas with a variety of possible toppings (chosen carefully by you, of course). They could make their own sandwiches in much the same way. Supply good ingredients, leave them to it, and you could be surprised at how much they eat – and at some of the rather unusual combinations.

🍽 Children can help with the weighing out of ingredients when you're following a recipe – and they won't notice that it's not far removed from maths!

🍽 They're quite handy too when you want help with the washing up of pots and pans. Children love sloshing about in water.

🍽 Children can help lay the table, because there are lots of things they are perfectly capable of, even at a very young age. They could lay out the knives, forks and spoons, they could fold napkins, fill jugs and glasses with water – even arrange some flowers in water for the centre of the table.

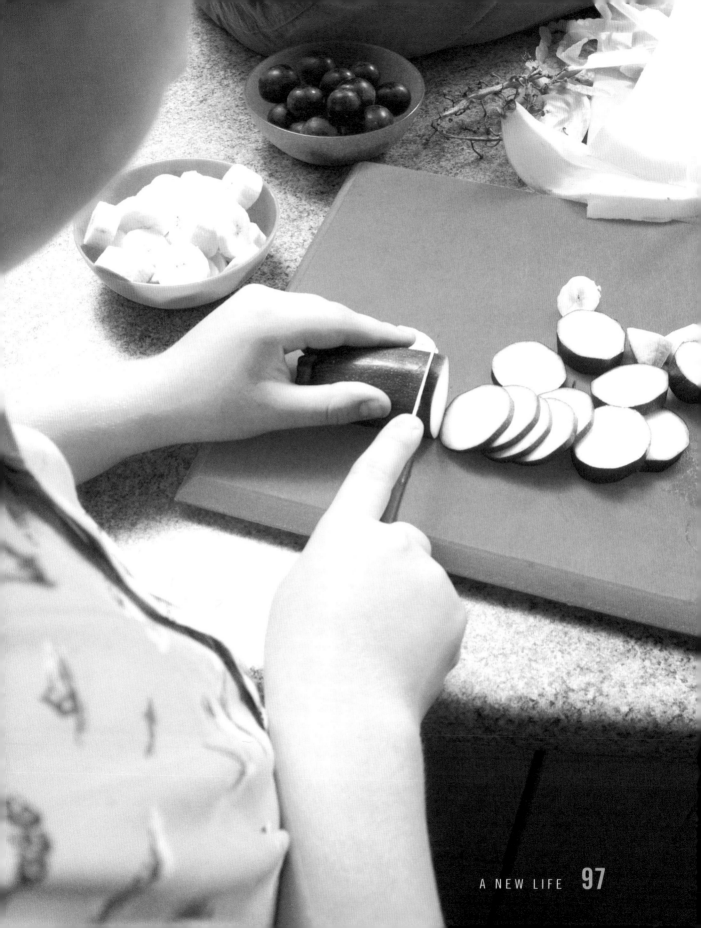

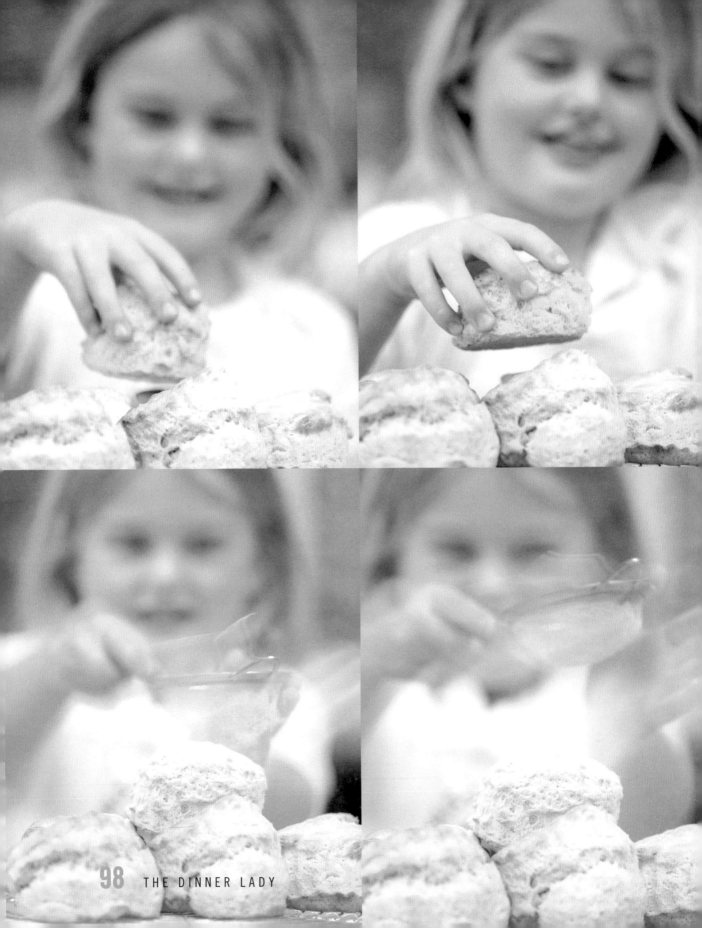

THE DINNER LADY

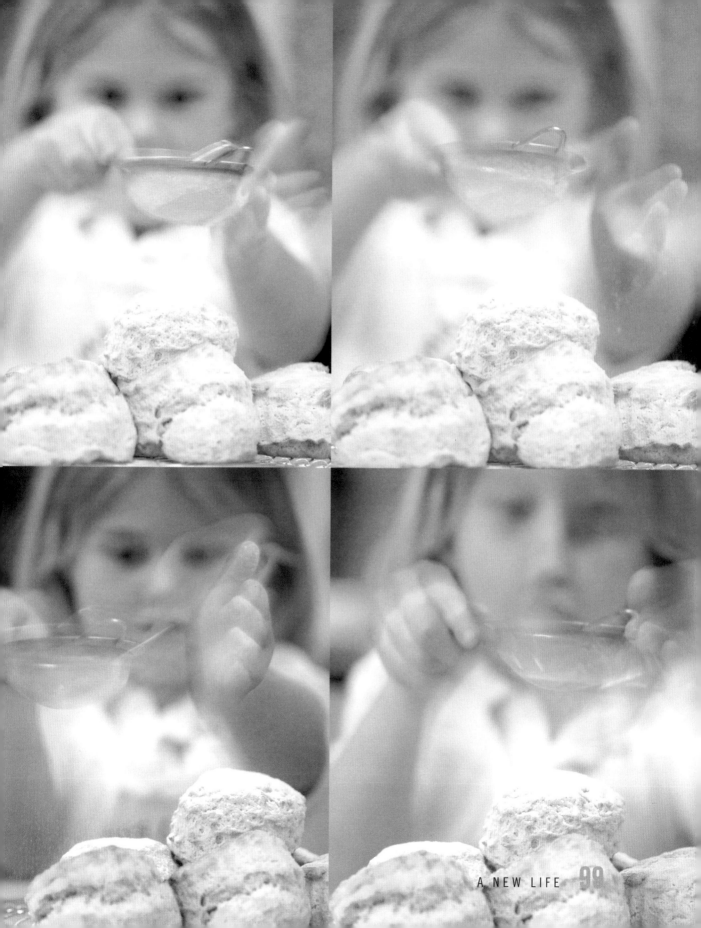

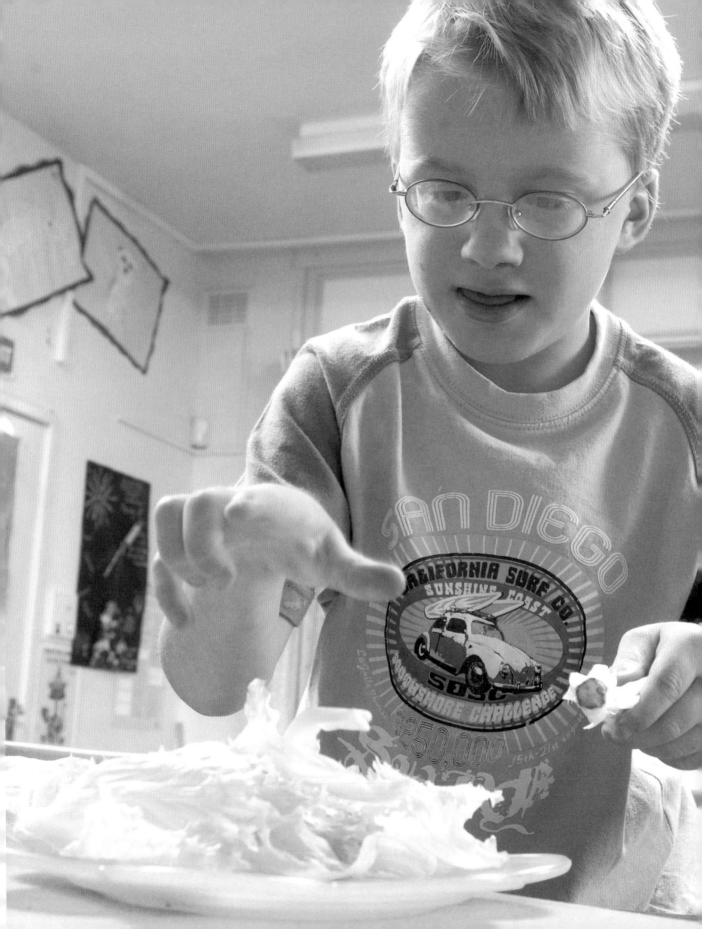

In the Public Eye

OUR WORK AT ST PETER'S suddenly started to come to the attention of the media, and this has been one of the most surprising aspects of my new life. It probably started in 2001 when I entered a competition called 'I Love My Cook' (sponsored by the British Meat & Livestock Commission) with a pasta dish I'd invented, using the new local bacon, which the kids loved. I submitted my entry with a short piece about St Peter's and a typical weekly menu. On the day of the competition I nervously cooked my pasta and followed it with a 'fruits of the forest shortbread'. I remember feeling all fingers and thumbs in a new and different kitchen, especially as it was divided into five sections, through which the judges wandered, checking and assessing. But the awards ceremony was fantastic. I was the runner-up – receiving '5 stars' – and returned to Nottinghamshire feeling very pleased with myself. Back in the kitchen I thought that was that and got on with my job as usual.

But things were never the same again. The commission issued a press release, and the phone started ringing. Not long afterwards, I was contacted by Friends of the Earth, who were holding a conference in Belfast. Would I be interested in talking about what we were doing at St Peter's? This was a challenge. I had never spoken in public before, and no one had ever previously been interested in what I thought about school meals. Anyway I wrote a speech (if you can call it that), forgot every word when I got to the conference hall, and just spoke from the heart. I found it very daunting, not least because I had never thought I would have the strength or the confidence to speak in public. However, because I believed so strongly in what I was about, I think I got my message across, and hopefully touched many nerves. I was then asked to write a piece for the Friends of the Earth magazine. Can you imagine how I felt – a dinner lady flying off to Belfast, speaking in front of a roomful of experts, and then being published in a national magazine!

After that first entry into public life, I remember thinking, 'Wow, my five minutes of fame!' before I got back to my kitchen. But it was just the start of a string of phone calls from newspapers, organizations and, closest to my heart, from schools. Heads, parents, governors and dinner ladies were all wanting advice about how they could do the same as we had been doing at St Peter's. One of the most significant calls was from a lady called Lizzie Vann. She, as I was later to discover, was an organics campaigner and founder of the Organix children's food company, as well as stepmother to three girls, and a governor of a school in Hampshire. She told me that she was very inspired by what we had achieved at St Peter's, and felt that more schools should follow suit. She invited me down to her primary school, Sopley Primary, near Christchurch. That was one of my first school excursions, and I was quite nervous.

But many similar requests started to come in, and I found myself travelling back and forth across the country, talking to primary schools. David was beginning to find this a little worrying. He was behind me every inch of the way, but I was on his payroll still, and I was always away, leaving much of the day-to-day work at St Peter's to the other ladies in the kitchen. Thus it was around this time that we dreamed up the idea of Primary Choice. Because I knew other dinner ladies could benefit from all I had experienced in the last couple of years, I thought a consulting company would be useful, showing other schools how they could source food locally, thereby cutting out food miles, helping the local economy and struggling local farmers, at the same time as allowing school cooks and kitchen assistants to rediscover and reuse their forgotten skills. The idea was that the schools needing help would actually *pay* for my services, which would help to balance David's books. I wrote a manifesto – I was becoming quite a dab hand at this by now – formed a company (with the school as my partner) and launched myself into business.

Primary Choice has been rather a success, and although my double life has been quite difficult – driving back from Totnes or Newcastle to don my dinner-lady pinny and make sure that St Peter's is still running smoothly – it is still going strong. (Now, though, because so many schools could not easily pay for the advice I was offering, the success of Primary Choice is due to my relationship with the Soil Association, of which more later.) I have been into school kitchens all over the country, talking to dinner ladies and teachers, watching what goes on in a multitude of schools, examining the contents of fridges and store cupboards, and generally giving advice on how to streamline and improve operations, how to access local suppliers, how to cost things properly, and how to set about going solo. This whole process must be taken slowly, something I have to instil in no uncertain terms into overenthusiastic dinner ladies or mothers wanting to bring about change at their school. In fact, for some smaller schools, this is not financially viable. So my advice has always been, if possible, to work with your local authority, as some are actually quite enlightened. I have been fortunate enough to work with Kay Knight of South Gloucestershire, where they are doing exactly what we are doing at St Peter's, but on a much greater scale, on a county level – and that involves no fewer than 119 schools.

We all want to rush into things and see instant results, but when you're dealing with councils, producers, elaborate costings and, not least, children with established and ingrained tastes, you have to accept that it's all going to take time.

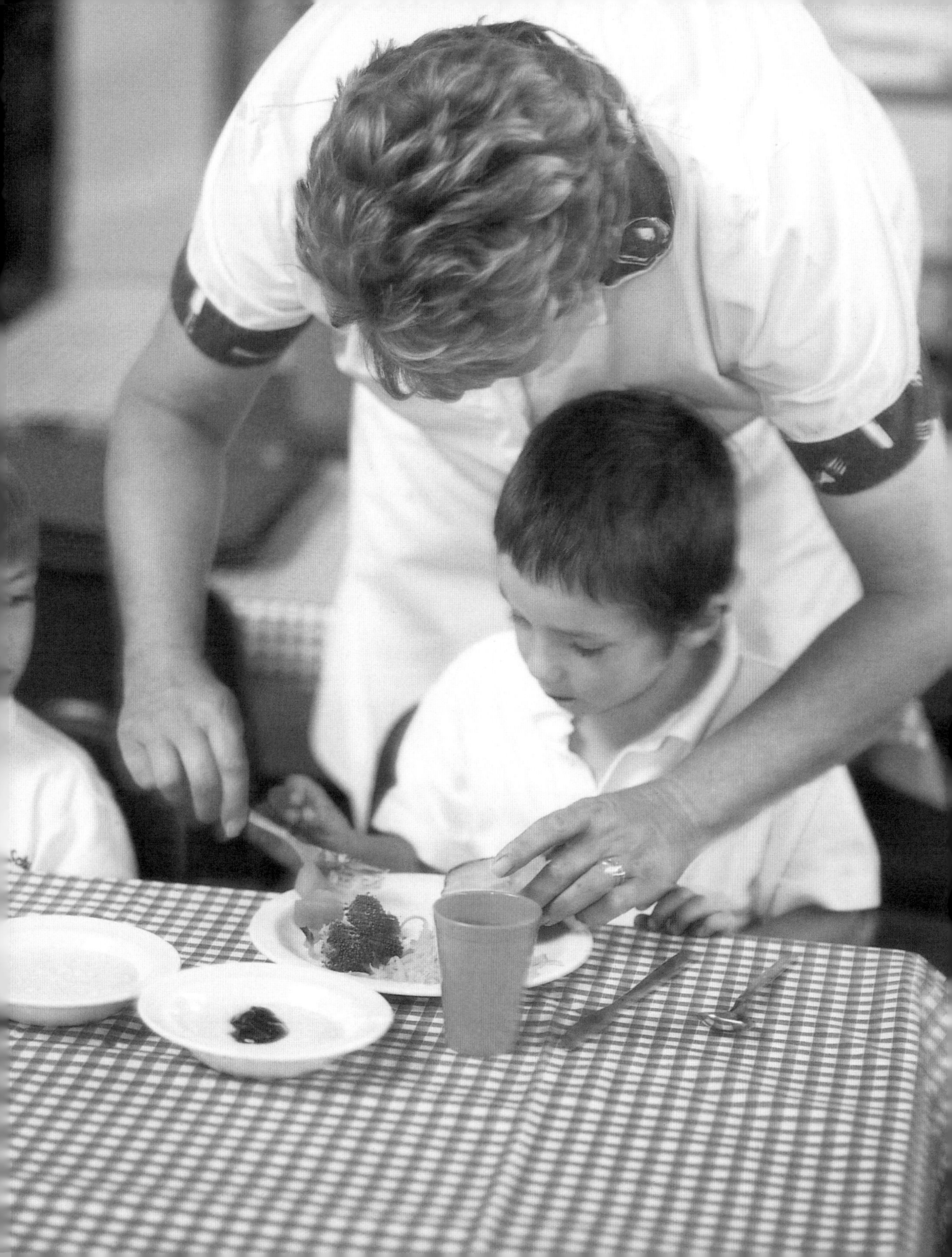

Food for Life

S**T PETER'S HAD A LETTER** in about mid-2002 from the Soil Association, asking if we would like to take part in what they called the 'Local Food Initiative of the year', part of the Soil Association Organic Food Awards 2002 (in tandem with *YOU* magazine). These awards had been running then for some seventeen years, working to honour growers and breeders who have done wonderful things in particular categories such as beer, wine, coffee, beef, pork, etc., and those who have excelled in other areas, such as restaurant of the year, or box scheme of the year. The only trouble was that our entry had to be put together and handed in within two weeks from when we received the letter. I got together with David – who, typically, said, 'No problem' – and we set about compiling an A4 folder describing what we had been doing, and containing some of our cuttings. I photocopied endlessly (we had to submit six copies for the judges), and wrote the intervening bits, while David composed a wonderful letter. When we hadn't heard anything for a while, me being me, I phoned up and spoke to Christopher Stopes, the Soil Association man who had contacted me before. 'What's happening?' asks I, and he said we were doing OK, but did we have any more material? I put together some more stuff, about the local milk if I remember, and sent it off by e-mail. Then on 12 September we heard that St Peter's School Catering Service was a joint winner nationwide in that Local Food Initiative category (sharing the prize with an organic fruit and vegetable distribution scheme in the Yorkshire Dales, called Growing with Grace).

Fancy being forty-six years old, and never having been to London before!

David and I went down to London for the lunch, on Friday 18 October, at the Dorchester. I was very excited as it was my first visit to London (fancy being forty-six years old, and never having been to London before!). The lunch was delicious, and awards were presented by the fashion designer Katherine Hamnett, Sue Peart, editor of *YOU* magazine, and Craig Sams, chairman of the Soil Association. There were so many well-known people there, who came and talked to us, that I was quite overwhelmed.

After that, everything went mad. I was in great demand. I was asked to meetings, presentations and to make speeches with organizations such as the Countryside Agency, the NFU (National Farmers' Union) and Defra (Department for Environment, Food and Rural Affairs). To follow were interviews with glossy women's magazines and radio appearances. I was asked by Sarah Brown, wife of the Chancellor of the Exchequer, to contribute to a

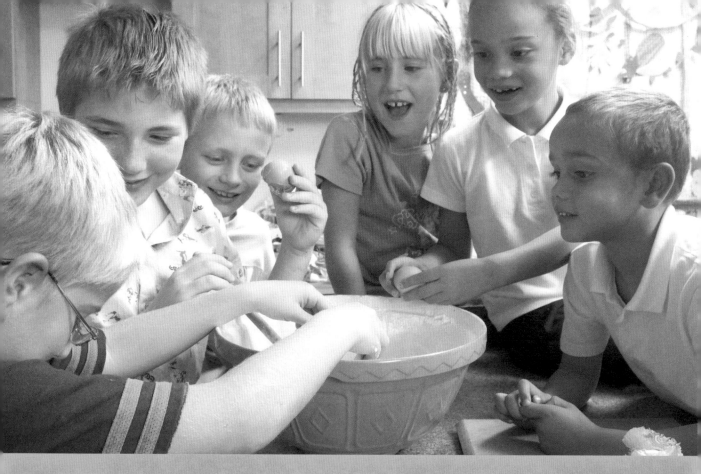

charity book she was editing. (I went to its launch at 11 Downing Street in April 2003, and found myself rubbing shoulders with Gary Rhodes, Richard Branson, David Frost and Nigel Havers – me, a dinner lady!) But one of the best things to come of that Soil Association day at the Dorchester was a renewal of my acquaintanceship with Lizzie Vann. After chatting there, we kept in touch on a regular basis, both of us passionate about improving food in schools, and both wondering what the next step might be. After meeting again at a Soil Association conference, we eventually decided we needed a report, something that would spill the beans about what school meals were really like, which would be very much based on the Primary Choice blueprint. Lizzie wanted to call it 'green' something, I seem to remember, while I was keener on the words 'food' and 'lifetime'.

With the help of Simon Brenman, a freelance consultant for organic producers and suppliers, we settled on the title 'Food for Life' – which, of course, is what it is all about. We then set about putting together a model that would advise schools or badger councils around the country on how to take control of their own school meal service. We contacted the Soil Association about our idea, and they took it on board with great enthusiasm. Lord Melchett, the policy director, and an organic farmer himself, and Patrick

Holden, the director, were very impressed with what we were trying to do. Thereafter they worked to get funding to publish the report (they are a charity, so couldn't back it themselves). Peter Melchett and his team made contact with the Calouste Gulbenkian Foundation to ask whether they would sponsor our proposed report. The Foundation agreed, and on 15 October 2003, the Food for Life report, written by Hannah Pearce, was launched. The basic message was simple, that most school lunches were of poor quality. The report urged the government (Department for Education and Skills, DfES) to take six key actions:

- It should establish national standards for school meals.

- It should provide sufficient new funding (at least double) for improved ingredients.

- It should adopt the Food for Life targets: that at least 30 per cent of the ingredients in the total number of school meals per week should be from certified organic sources, that at least 50 per cent of the ingredients should be sourced locally from the region, and that 75 per cent of all food eaten should be prepared from unprocessed ingredients.

- DfES and LEAs should aim for 100 per cent uptake of school meals within ten years.

- Parents, children and teachers should be involved in the planning of school meals, and all should eat together regularly in order to emphasize the idea of meals being sociable, pleasant and even educational times.

- Children should be encouraged to learn about food and the food chain in all relevant aspects of the school curriculum.

Accompanying the report was a press release that really set the cat among the pigeons. Headlines screamed out: 'The 31p lunch that may make pupils ill' (*The Times*) and 'Children are served "cheap muck in schools"' (*Independent*). One of the revelations that attracted all this attention was that the daily amount spent on a child's school lunch could be as low as 31p, compared with around 60p spent on lunch for someone in prison. (To this day I am dubious about this comment, because an adult in prison usually has twice the body weight, at least, of a child. It was an unfair comparison, I think, and the hysteria was a little unjustified.) It was Peter Melchett who coined the phrase 'muck off a truck' to describe the low-quality and low-price processed foods, such as breaded fish or chicken shapes, that were dominating the school dinners served by contract caterers. I have come to know Peter Melchett very well, and this was in no way a slur on dinner ladies themselves, more a condemnation of the food they were being forced to serve.

A BRIEF INTRODUCTION TO THE SOIL ASSOCIATION

THE SOIL ASSOCIATION IS AN INDEPENDENT, not-for-profit organization, and one of the UK's most respected environmental groups. The inspiration behind the organization was a book by Lady Eve Balfour, *The Living Soil*, published in 1943; this presented the case for an alternative approach to the intensive farming methods then in force (and this alternative approach has since become known as organic farming).

Three years later, in 1946, a group of farmers, scientists and nutritionists founded the Soil Association, and since then it has campaigned for safer, healthier food and sustainable agriculture, based on the connection between healthy soil, healthy food and healthy people. The association has developed organic standards and now works with consumers, farmers, growers, retailers and policy makers. It is also the largest UK organic certification body, and certifies over 70 per cent of UK licensed producers and processors.

To quote them, 'Healthy food means a healthy you. This is why we believe that agriculture is the primary health service.'

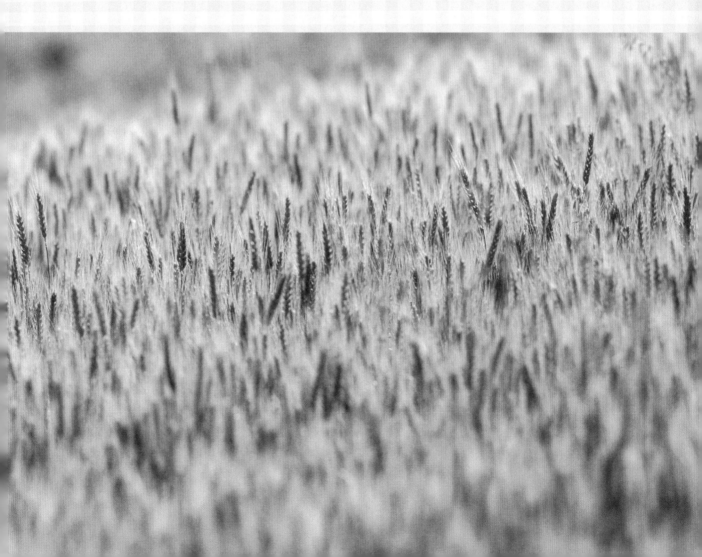

In the report, an analysis of primary school menus showed that the same trends dominating the supermarkets and displacing fresh food from home kitchens were eroding the quality of school meals. Regardless of the healthy eating messages promoted in the classroom, most school dinner menus were dominated by cheap processed and fast-food items packed with fat, salt and refined sugar, laden with artificial flavourings, colourings or preservatives, and precariously low in essential nutrients. This was very close to my heart, as there doesn't seem to be much point in telling children to eat healthily – the 'Five a Day' and other health messages around – when what they were eating at school was possibly the least healthy option they could get.

The report demanded that government nutritional standards for school meals should be set and closely monitored; these had been removed, of course, after the 1980 Education Act. The report's recommendation that the amount of money spent on ingredients should be doubled was important because it had long been acknowledged that poor diet led to increased illness, and to obesity. Lizzie Vann was quoted as saying, 'The declining quality of school meals is creating a public-health time-bomb', which is undoubtedly true: diet-related illness is a greater problem than smoking, apparently, costing the NHS at least £2.5 billion every year. This too was central to my own thinking. I had started off wanting my children at St Peter's to eat healthily, but the picture was becoming even bigger. With the recommendations in the report, perhaps we could influence people to start their children off on the right diets from the beginning. If parents offered a variety of good foods right from the start of weaning, then the children would be naturally inclined towards good foods once they went to school – so long as the schools were enabled to serve good food. If they were familiar with the flavours of proper food, they would

LINKS BETWEEN FOOD AND BEHAVIOUR

TEACHERS IN SECONDARY SCHOOLS HAVE TOLD me about kids having problems in the afternoon after a lunch consisting of chocolate, crisps and fizzy drinks from the vending machines. All the sugar makes them as high as a kite, but within as short a time as twenty minutes, this can dissipate, meaning they come down from their high, get grumpy and hungry, and can't concentrate as a result.

That good food and behaviour are linked is not now disputed. A special school in the north of England noted that children with autism visibly and enduringly altered in behaviour when their diet was changed to one omitting wheat, and including lots of fruit and vegetables. A study of young prison inmates in Buckinghamshire found that feeding them fresh vegetables rather than processed foods helped to cut the number of offences by more than a quarter. The number of violent incidents also fell by more than 40 per cent. Children fed on a 'wartime' diet (see page 59) were also noticeably calmer than the ones on a contemporary fat- and sugar-rich diet.

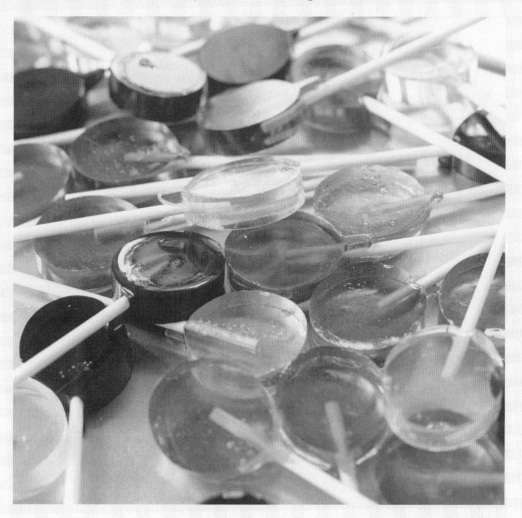

react against the artificial saltiness and sweetness of processed foods. At the end of 2004, the government brought out a Healthy Living Blueprint, in which they announced that they were going to initiate changes in secondary schools, and consider primary and nursery schools later. That is completely wrong thinking to me. Secondary school is far too late, and they are starting at the wrong end.

Reactions to the Food for Life report continued to dominate the press. The *Guardian* challenged three chefs and a nutritionist to come up with a good healthy meal, spending the same 31p that was quoted above. Raymond Blanc, whom I had met earlier at a Soil Association workshop in Cirencester, was one of them. He had asked me to come to a meal at his Le Manoir aux Quat'Saisons, but I had to turn him down. (I had a meeting with Nottinghamshire County Council, but ask me again, Raymond!) He suggested polenta made with milk, cheese, egg and a vegetable such as peas, followed by baked apple rolled in sugar and cinnamon, or a crème caramel. Giorgio Locatelli suggested lasagne, beans and cereal, and said that in Italy they spent 96p per head, and just over £1 in France – I wish. (He was later quoted in the *Daily Mail*: 'What you put in the mouths of your children is more important than what you put on their bodies or in their brains. I cannot believe we exist in a society that says it cares about children, yet fails to teach them what is good to eat.' Music to my ears.) The River Café chefs, Rose Grey and Ruth Rogers, suggested a risotto and a baked pear, and Kate Harrod-Wild, the nutritionist, a sandwich, jacket potato or stir-fry. All of these professionals found it very difficult indeed to come up with something nutritious for that amount of money, so I hope the message was getting across to those that mattered.

> 'What you put in the mouths of your children is more important than what you put on their bodies or in their brains'.

Soon after the launch date, the Soil Association became inundated with requests for further information and help from schools around the UK. The impact of the report exceeded their expectations and they didn't have the manpower to deal with the response, so they sought further monetary help from the Calouste Gulbenkian Foundation to employ me for two days a week. I couldn't believe it! I was asked to visit and meet with schools far and wide to help upgrade their catering systems in line with the Food for Life model, which tied in, of course, with Primary Choice. And that wasn't all. I was also asked to help with higher levels of policy, to meet with officials and ministers, to attend conferences and meetings with MPs and Local Authority School Meals Providers as well as other dinner ladies and unions. Lord (Larry) Whitty, Minister for Food, Farming and Sustainable Energy, visited the school in November 2003 (just before we were both to speak at a Public Sector Food

Procurement Conference). He had lunch with the children, and we served him roast lamb, roast potatoes, broccoli and carrots. For the children an even more exciting visitor was Jamie Oliver, who came to discuss good food and school dinners, and to film for a new television series. And meanwhile, I was winner of the BBC Radio 4 Food and Farming Awards for Best Public Caterer, 2003, and the Observer Food Award for 'Person who has done the most for the food and drink industry in 2003'. I went to Highgrove to meet Prince Charles, and in September 2004, I was elected Midlands Woman of Achievement by the Winged Fellowship Trust.

It may be a bit overwhelming, but I am doing something that I love. So, with me out of the kitchen twice a week, we had to make some changes at St Peter's. We promoted Christine to cook-in-charge, Alison moved up to assist Christine, Jane was promoted into her position as kitchen assistant and we employed another Christine to help. I know St Peter's is in very safe hands.

And the Future?

M Y PRINCIPAL HOPE IS that government, LEAs, schools, private catering companies and parents will be able to take on board and implement all the suggestions of the Food for Life report. But I have many other visions of how we can continue to change the way our children eat.

At St Peter's – and at many other schools now throughout the country – food and the concept of healthy eating is being incorporated into the curriculum in a number of ways. Government and other bodies are behind several ideas such as the National Fruit Scheme (key stage 1 children getting a free piece of fruit at break-time, a great idea), the Growing Schools Initiative (gardens and/or allotments attached to schools, where pupils can grow, tend and learn), Focus on Food (a food learning programme backed by the Royal Society of Arts and Waitrose), and Adopt a Pumpkin (another, smaller, growing initiative, run by Ashlyns Organic Farm in Essex – a farm, incidentally, which has become very important for schools in that part of the country). The Academy of Culinary Arts provides chefs who are willing to 'adopt a school' and provide culinary inspiration to pupils, and the Guild of Food Writers has a Cook It! campaign to spread the word among children that food and cooking are fun. Many famous and successful chefs have started to involve themselves: Jamie Oliver for one, and Gordon Ramsay, who went to a primary school in London to cook dinner.

Many famous and successful chefs have started to involve themselves: Jamie Oliver for one …

But it is the loss of cooking on the school curriculum that most upsets me. The old domestic science classes were not wonderful (I disliked them intensely), but with cooking being subsumed into Design and Technology in 1992, the majority of young people are not learning a fundamental life skill. A whole generation (almost two now) is growing up without learning about nutrition, food and the basics of home cooking. It is food illiteracy. Educationalists may believe that the GCSE Food Technology course is more relevant in today's world, but in reality the course is more about how the food industry operates. It is more theoretical than practical, and children learn, I believe, how to design a box for pizza, rather than learn how to design a pizza to eat. This is echoed by food writer Sue Style in an article in *Waitrose Food Illustrated*: '…"food technology", where pupils are asked to "evaluate a variety of ready-prepared meals", "modify a pie" or "design and make food products" (no mention of "dishes", "meals", or even "cooking").' The emphasis is completely wrong, and I believe we should be backtracking and reintroducing basic kitchen skills and knowledge. There are some dedicated cookery schools for children (the Kids' Cookery School in West London teaches more than 2000 children to cook per year), but it is government that should introduce a coherent food programme. Cooking is, after all, an enjoyable experience, something families can do together, and so much more satisfying than shoving ready meals into the microwave – what my husband calls 'ping dinners'! Even if they do it only at weekends, it's got to be better than not doing it at all. It's also more nutritious – and cheaper.

Food advertising is another of my bugbears. During World War Two, the Ministry of Food, with the aid of Marguerite Patten, encouraged the eating of vegetables by inventing characters like 'Dr Carrot, the children's friend', and 'Potato Pete'. These were enticing ideas, rather than hectoring (eat five a day, or else), and I am sure we could be more imaginative about making good foods more attractive. Sadly, it is principally 'bad' foods like cakes, biscuits and sweets that have most advertising money spent on them – you never see the same enthusiasm applied to carrots, peas or Brussels sprouts. If David Beckham advertised carrots, then carrots would probably shoot up in popularity, so much so that the farmers might not be able to produce enough! Children's heroes, both fictional cartoon and real-life, could be used very successfully to sell spinach or broccoli, rather than the undesirable foods they now sponsor. And the interconnection between commercial food companies and schools makes my blood boil. Vending machines in secondary schools are put there by big companies to sell their crisps, sweets and fizzy drinks. In most cases the school will agree because some of the income from the machines is permitted to be retained by the school – and this is often how schools pay for that extra teacher. Saving empty packets of crisps or chocolate wrappers in exchange for school sports equipment, and other such advertising schemes, are in the same distasteful arena. Schools should never have to sink to those levels, especially when the health of children is at stake. One of Food for Life's targets is to get more government money for school-dinner ingredients. Another vision would be to get more government money for schools, full stop.

Another subject I am passionate about is the status of dinner ladies, cooks and kitchen assistants. They work long hours, for very little pay, and are often forgotten about. (I have worked in schools, for instance, where teachers did not speak to me, as my job was obviously considered beneath their notice.) But the ladies in a school kitchen (and they are mostly ladies) are responsible for feeding the next generation. They are looking after one of the most high-risk groups in the country, children, and are also responsible for giving them a meal that constitutes a third of their daily intake (sometimes, sadly, it can be the main meal of the day). They are often considered to be unskilled, but running a school kitchen demands certain national and county requirements: you have to know about health and safety, have acquired hygiene certificates (I have intermediate and advanced, as well as one in training), and numerous other, rather arcane, specialities (hazard analysis, critical control points, etc.). Actually, a passion for cooking is a major basic! But catering is the only trade where, if something goes wrong, you are guilty until proven innocent, and the bottom line, which I now emphasize wherever I go, is that we can kill. So dinner ladies need to know what they are doing, and I think they ought to be recognized for their skills and dedication. Numbers may have diminished following the 1980 Education Act and many skilled people may have been lost (when all we had to do was scissor open packets), but we need now to encourage the best people back into the business. Rose Grey, of the River Café in London, founded a charity called Cooks in Schools in 2004, and one of its proposed aims is to help train school cooks. I'm all in favour of that. And I should also like to institute a cooks' or dinner ladies' conference, held annually, so that we can all get together and talk about what is happening in schools and school kitchens. Dinner ladies form an integral part of the society that is a school, and their role ought to be acknowledged more publicly.

I have worked in schools, for instance, where teachers did not speak to me, as my job was obviously considered beneath their notice.

And, although I may only be one of those self-same school dinner ladies, I am one who wants to make a difference. This generation of children has been called the 'Chicken Nugget Generation', but I want it to be the last to be fed such rubbish. I have met thousands of parents, teachers, cooks and school governors over the past few years as I have travelled up and down the country visiting schools, and I know there is a passion out there for good food. People worry about cooking being too complicated, or time-consuming. It doesn't have to be either, and whether you're at home or in a school kitchen, I hope my book inspires you to give it a go …

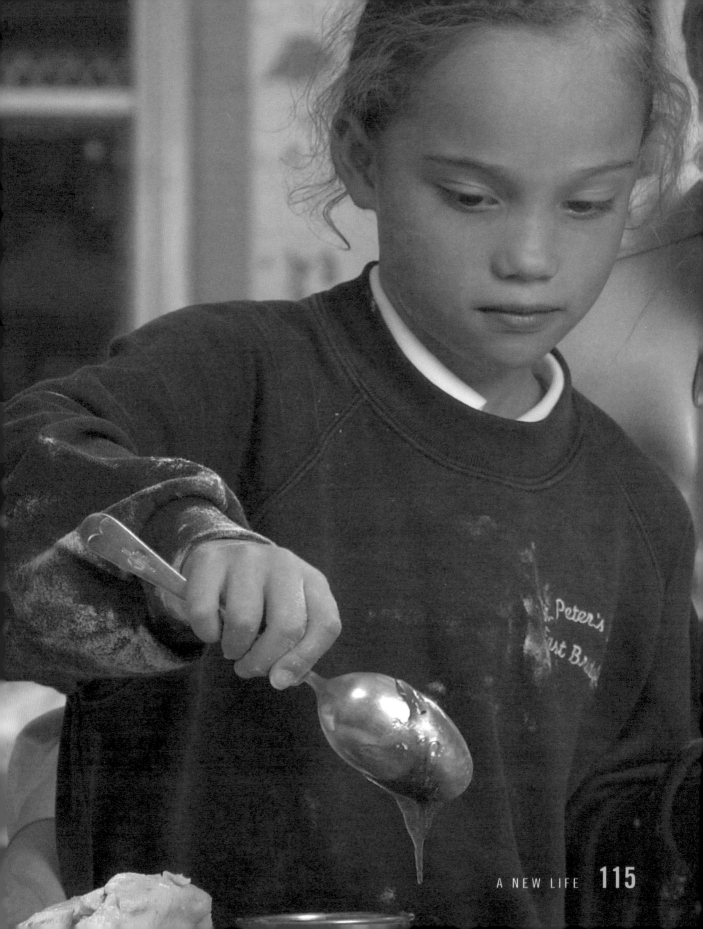

SEASONAL FOODS CHART

	SPRING (March, April, May)	SUMMER (June, July, August)
Vegetables	Asparagus, avocado pears, beetroot, broad beans, cabbage, carrots, cauliflower, celeriac, chicory, leeks, parsnips, potatoes (new), purple-sprouting broccoli, radishes, sea kale, shallots, sorrel, spinach, spring greens, spring onions, swedes, turnips, watercress	Asparagus, aubergines, beetroot, broad beans, broccoli, cabbage, capsicums, carrots, cauliflower, courgettes, cucumbers, globe artichokes, green beans, lettuces, mangetout, peas, potatoes (new), radishes, spinach, spring onions, sweetcorn, tomatoes, watercress
Fruit and nuts	Bananas, Cape gooseberries, citrus fruits, pineapples, rhubarb	Apricots, bilberries, blackberries, blackcurrants, blueberries, cherries, gooseberries, grapes, loganberries, mangoes, melons, nectarines, peaches, plums, raspberries, redcurrants, strawberries, whitecurrants
Fish	Brill, cod, coley, conger eel, crab, crawfish, flounder, haddock, halibut, lemon sole, lobster, mackerel, salmon, sea trout, whitebait	Crab, Dover sole, grey mullet, haddock, hake, halibut, herring, lobster, plaice, prawns, salmon, sardines, sea bass, sea bream, sea trout, shrimps, squid
Meat	Beef, chicken, lamb, pork	Beef, chicken, guinea fowl, lamb

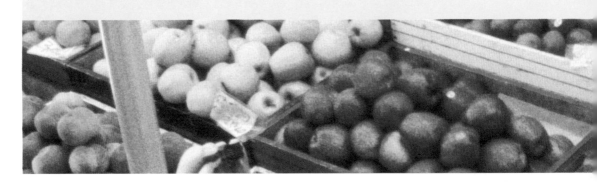

AUTUMN (September, October, November)	WINTER (December, January, February)	
Aubergines, beetroot, broccoli, capsicums, carrots, cauliflower, celeriac, celery, courgettes, fennel, green beans, kohlrabi, leeks, marrows and squashes, onions, parsnips, pumpkins, swedes, sweet potatoes, turnips	Avocado pears, beetroot, chicory, Brussels sprouts, cabbage (red and Savoy), carrots, celeriac, kale, chard, sea kale, shallots, fennel, Jerusalem artichokes, kohlrabi, leeks, onions, parsnips, potatoes (old), pumpkins, sweet potatoes, turnips	**Vegetables**
Almonds, apples, blackberries, Brazil nuts, chestnuts, crab apples, cranberries, damsons, dates, citrus fruits, figs, grapes, hazelnuts, pears, plums, pomegranates, quinces, walnuts	Almonds, apples, Brazil nuts, Cape gooseberries, chestnuts, citrus fruits, cranberries, dates, grapes, lychees, mangoes, pears, pineapples, pomegranates, rhubarb, walnuts	**Fruit and nuts**
Carp, cod, coley, conger eel, Dover sole, eel, grey mullet, haddock, hake, halibut, herring, huss, ling, mackerel, pilchards, plaice, prawns, sea bass, sea bream, shrimps, skate, squid, turbot	Carp, cod, coley, conger eel, Dover sole, eel, grey mullet, haddock, hake, halibut, herring, huss, lemon sole, ling, mackerel, mussels, plaice, sea bass, sea bream, skate, turbot, whiting	**Fish**
Beef, chicken, duck, goose, grouse, guinea fowl, hare, partridge, pheasant, pigeon, pork, rabbit, venison	Beef, chicken, duck (farmed and wild), goose, guinea fowl, hare, pheasant, pigeon, pork, rabbit, turkey, venison	**Meat**

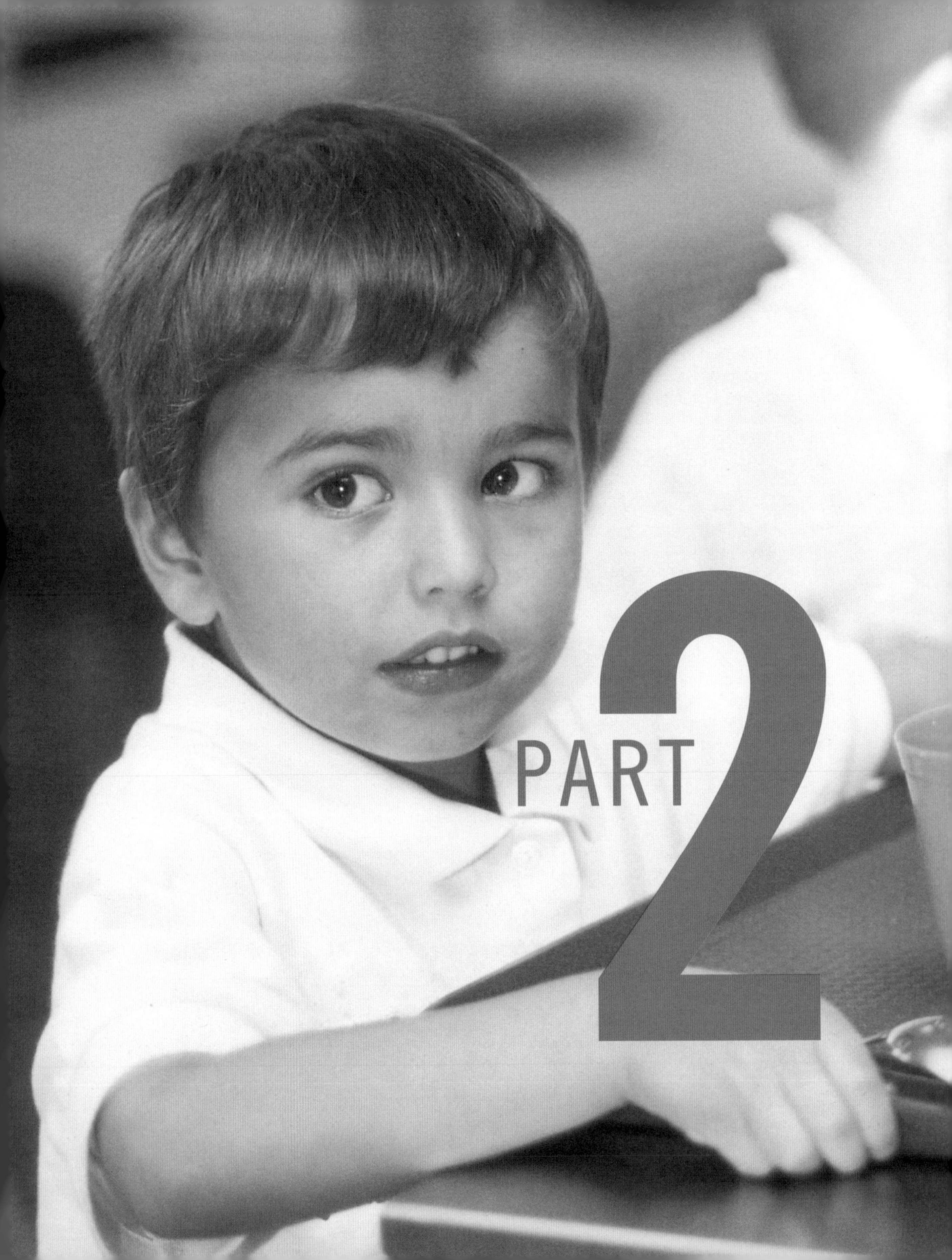

PART 2

School Dinner Recipes

*A*LL THE RECIPES ARE FOR FOUR ADULTS AND 96 CHILDREN. *If you are cooking for children alone, the four adult portions would feed eight. And my quantities are generous …*

The method instructions are given for those cooking at home for four, as I am sure dinner ladies will know perfectly well how to adapt the formula for their greater numbers.

I have rarely added salt and pepper to any of the recipes, as I think these should be used as sparingly as possible.

Never pile too much of a main course on a child's plate. You don't want to 'out-face' them. If they have a small portion to start with, you never know, they might come back for more.

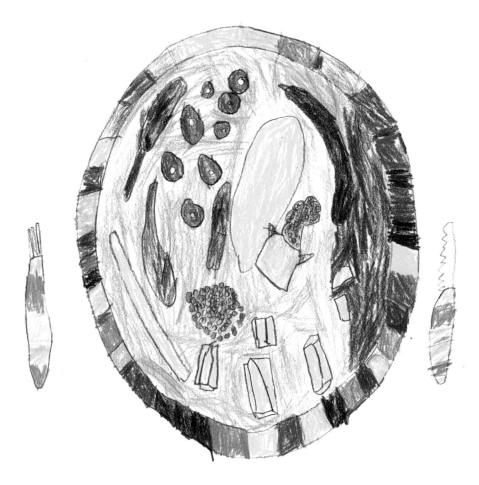

T HE MAIN COURSE lies at the heart of any lunch, whether at home or at school, for it is here that you can combine protein, carbohydrate, minerals and vitamins in good proportions to keep the children going throughout the afternoon.

Proteins are very important for children, because they are needed by the body during periods of growth. Some proteins are 'complete' (such as milk, meat, poultry, fish, eggs, cheese and yoghurt), while some are what is known as 'incomplete' (grains and all things made from them, such as bread, cereals and pasta, as well as pulses, nuts and seeds). Sometimes a combination of the two – macaroni with cheese, spaghetti bolognaise, cereal with milk – can be as nutritious as, and cheaper than, a good cut of meat.

Meat, whether white (poultry) or red (lamb, beef or pork), should be sourced locally, and have been raised organically if at all possible. I have a wonderful local butcher who produces meat to careful specification, as we have no time in the school kitchen to trim, chop and mince. If I want lamb diced for a stew, that is what I order and what I get, already trimmed, with no wastage.

Fish is rich in protein and minerals, easy to digest and very easy to cook, but I am finding it increasingly difficult to source. Organically speaking, fish presents a problem, for the EU has stated that nothing that is either captured or harvested from the wild can be called organic. The logic is obvious: organic food is about production, and wild food isn't 'produced'. Some farmed fish can be classified as organic, however. So far they include only salmon and sea trout, but I have heard that cod, halibut and sea bass are coming. When you buy wild fish caught at sea, do choose those that are not on an endangered list; the 'sustainability' issue that is so central to good food principles is particularly crucial when applied to wild food from the sea.

The commonest complaint amongst parents of primary-school-aged children must be that they don't eat vegetables. Quite why children should traditionally dislike them so much, I don't know – do they dislike the texture (for we famously overcook vegetables in the UK) or the colour (what's wrong with green food)? I certainly encountered some degree of resistance when I was transforming the menu at St Peter's, but I persevered, and now my children, without prompting, help themselves happily from a daily variety of hot dishes, and from the salad bar.

Colour I think is important, and the brightest coloured vegetables seem to be the most popular: sweetcorn, peas, green beans, broccoli, beetroot, tomatoes, carrots and red and yellow peppers. Cabbage and Brussels sprouts are less successful; because they are brassicas, they have a stronger taste, which is perhaps less attractive to younger palates. Shape and size is significant as well. I always cut broccoli, for instance, into small florets, which are more accessible to small eyes and mouths; I also cut carrots into different shapes, such as cubes, chunks, slices or sticks. And of course the cooking is the most important of all. The texture has to be just right – not too al dente, and certainly not too soft.

Most vegetables and fruits can be sourced locally and seasonally; always go for organic if possible. Some tastes that children like cannot be grown or bought locally, such as the banana and lemon used in some of the salads. When buying these warm-climate fruit, try to find Fairtrade produce. Fairtrade operates first on a basis of protecting its staff (safety, no forced child labour, maternity leave, fair wages etc.), but then starts to move towards the organic, with protection of the environment, bans on herbicides etc. Some Fairtrade producers still use some pesticides, but there is a worldwide movement towards pesticide reduction, followed by organic production and biological control if possible.

The egg and cheese dishes here are suitable for vegetarians, for whom eggs and cheese are prime sources of the 'complete' proteins that are a valuable element of their diet. Among the vegetable and salad dishes are accompanying dishes as well as satisfying main courses that are also suitable for vegetarians.

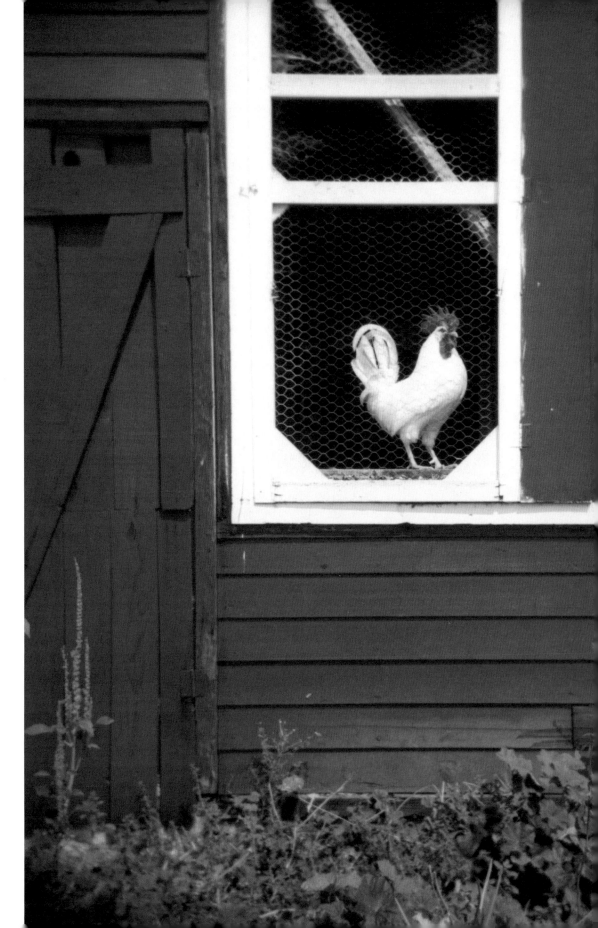

Chicken and Turkey

Chicken Curry

The older children like curry, and chicken is their favourite. You can add more curry powder to taste, or reduce the quantity. I make a very mild curry. You could also add some more vegetables, such as sweet potatoes, sliced peppers, even chickpeas from a can.

Serves 4		Serves 96
225g (8oz)	carrots	2.7kg (6lb)
225g (8oz)	onions	2.7kg (6lb)
1	garlic clove	5
225g (8oz)	eating apples	2.7kg (6lb)
1 tablespoon	lemon juice	2 tablespoons
1 tablespoon	olive oil	175ml (6fl oz)
1 tablespoon	mild curry powder	12 tablespoons
2 teaspoons	turmeric	4 tablespoons
450g (1lb)	diced chicken	5.4kg (12lb)
25g (1oz)	plain flour	350g (12oz)
600ml (1 pint)	water	6.8 litres (12 pints)
55g (2oz)	sultanas	600g (1lb 5oz)
1 tablespoon	mango chutney	350g (12oz)

If the carrots are new season, you can just give them a good wash, otherwise peel them; dice them quite small. Peel the onions, and roughly dice. Peel the garlic and finely chop. Peel and core the apples, then cut into quarters and dice. Leave them in the lemon juice so they will not go brown.

Put the onions in a saucepan with the olive oil, and cook over a moderate heat until soft. Add the garlic, carrot, curry powder and turmeric, and cook for a further 10 minutes or until the carrots are soft. Add the chicken, stir all the ingredients together, and cook for about 5 minutes to seal the chicken. Mix the flour and water together until smooth, then sieve into the mixture. Stir together well, then cover and cook for a further 30–35 minutes.

During the last 10 minutes of cooking, add the apples, sultanas and mango chutney to the chicken mixture, and mix. Serve with brown rice and naan bread.

Chicken Meatballs with Fresh Tomato Sauce

Another winner with the children at school, and so much better than out of a can. You could also use tomato passata instead of the fresh tomatoes in the sauce. And the sauce would be delicious served simply with pasta and grated Parmesan cheese.

Serves 4		Serves 96
450g (1lb)	minced chicken	*5.4kg (12lb)*
115g (4oz)	Cheddar cheese	*1.3kg (3lb)*
1	egg	*12*
115g (4oz)	white breadcrumbs	*1.3kg (3lb)*
2 teaspoons	dried mixed herbs	*115g (4oz)*
2 tablespoons	olive oil	*350ml (12fl oz)*
	Fresh tomato sauce	
1	onion	*12*
1.8kg (4lb)	tomatoes	*10.8kg (24lb)*
1 tablespoon	olive oil	*175ml (6fl oz)*
1 teaspoon	dried mixed herbs	*55g (2oz)*

To make the tomato sauce, first peel and slice the onion finely. Chop the tomatoes. Heat the oil in a large pan, add the onion and cook until soft. Add the tomatoes and mixed herbs, cover with a lid and bring to the boil, stirring occasionally. Reduce the heat to low, partially cover the pan with a lid, and cook gently for about 1 hour. At this stage sieve the tomato sauce to get rid of the skins.

Meanwhile, put the chicken into a bowl. Grate the cheese, and beat the egg. Add the cheese, egg, breadcrumbs and mixed herbs to the chicken, and mix well. Shape the mixture into about 16 balls and chill for 30 minutes in the fridge.

Heat the oil in a shallow pan and fry the balls in batches until brown on all sides. (If you are doing a large number, brown them in the oven in a greased tin at 180°C/350°F/Gas 4.)

Add the meatballs to the sauce and simmer without a lid for 20 minutes.

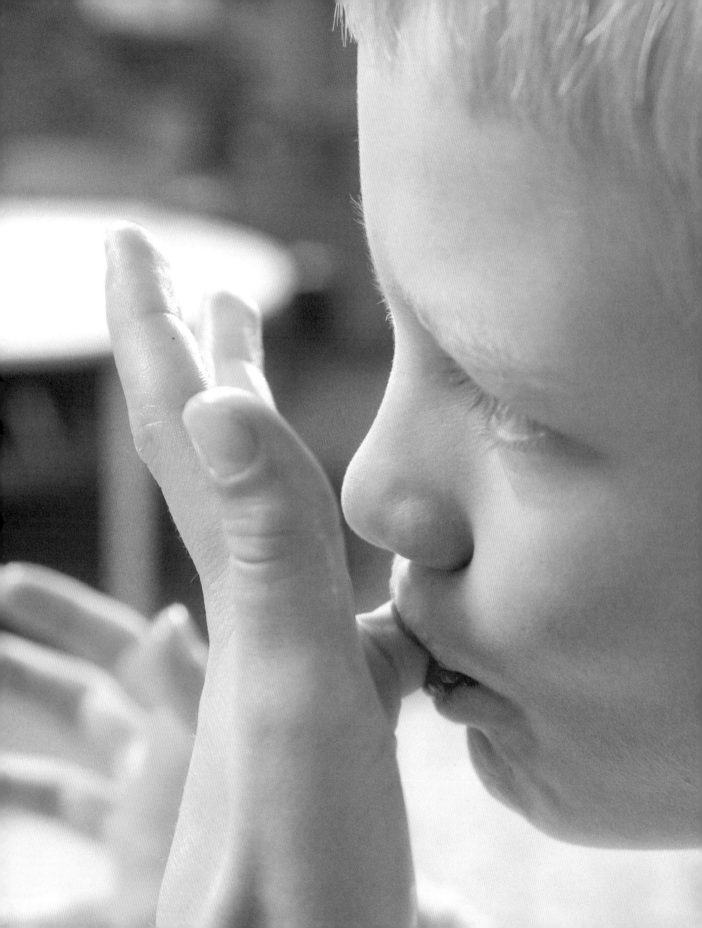

Tom's Sweet and Sour Chicken

You can make this with pork, turkey or chicken, but chicken seems to be the favourite every time. Kids love the sweet and sour flavours. Tom Crossland invented this recipe when we asked Year 5 to design a healthy menu.

Serves 4		Serves 96
115g (4oz)	onions	*1.3kg (3lb)*
175g (6oz)	carrots	*2kg (4½lb)*
1	red pepper	*12*
1 x 200g can	pineapple chunks in juice	*12 x 200g cans*
450g (1lb)	diced chicken	*5.4kg (12lb)*
25ml (1fl oz)	vegetable oil	*350ml (12fl oz)*
300ml (10fl oz)	water	*3.4 litres (6 pints)*
25g (1oz)	caster sugar	*300g (10½oz)*
25ml (1fl oz)	soy sauce	*350ml (12fl oz)*
40ml (1½fl oz)	vinegar	*500ml (18fl oz)*
115g (4oz)	tomato purée	*1.3kg (3lb)*
½ teaspoon	mustard powder	*25g (1oz)*
20g (¾oz)	cornflour	*250g (9oz)*
	To serve	
4–8	tortilla wraps	*96*

Peel and slice the onions and the carrots finely, and seed and slice the pepper. Drain the pineapple, reserving the juice.

Fry the chicken in the oil in batches until brown, then remove from the pan. Fry the onion, carrot and pepper until softened. Return the chicken to the pan, and add the pineapple juice and the water, along with the sugar, soy sauce, vinegar, tomato purée and mustard. Simmer for approximately 10 minutes, or until the chicken is tender.

Add the pineapple pieces. Blend the cornflour with a little water, and add to the mixture. Stir over the heat until the sauce thickens and the pineapple is warm. We serve the tortilla wrap separately on the side of the plate, with broccoli as the vegetable.

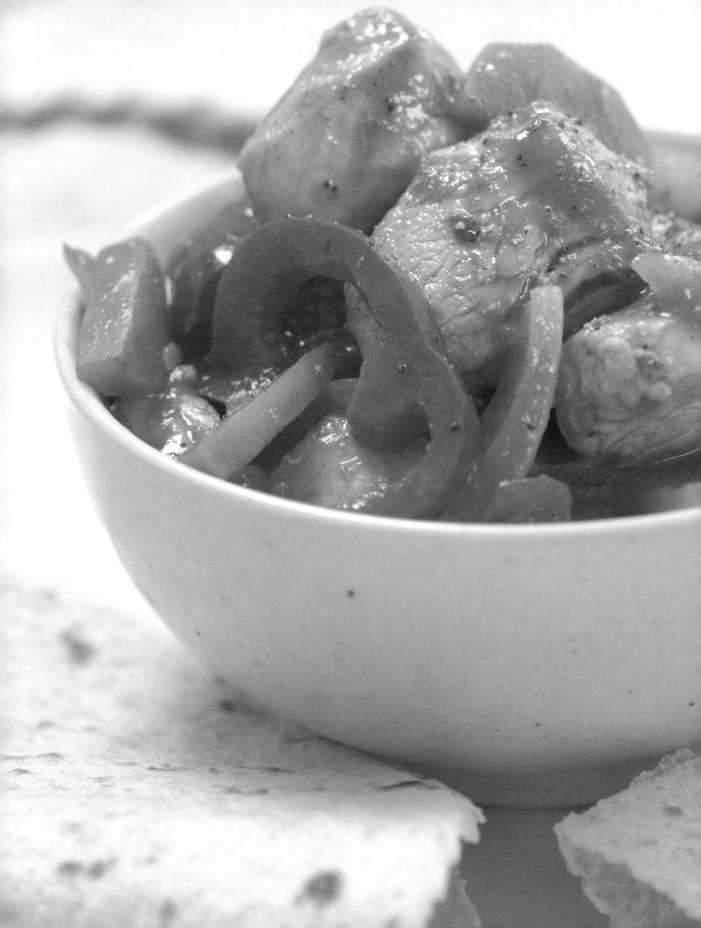

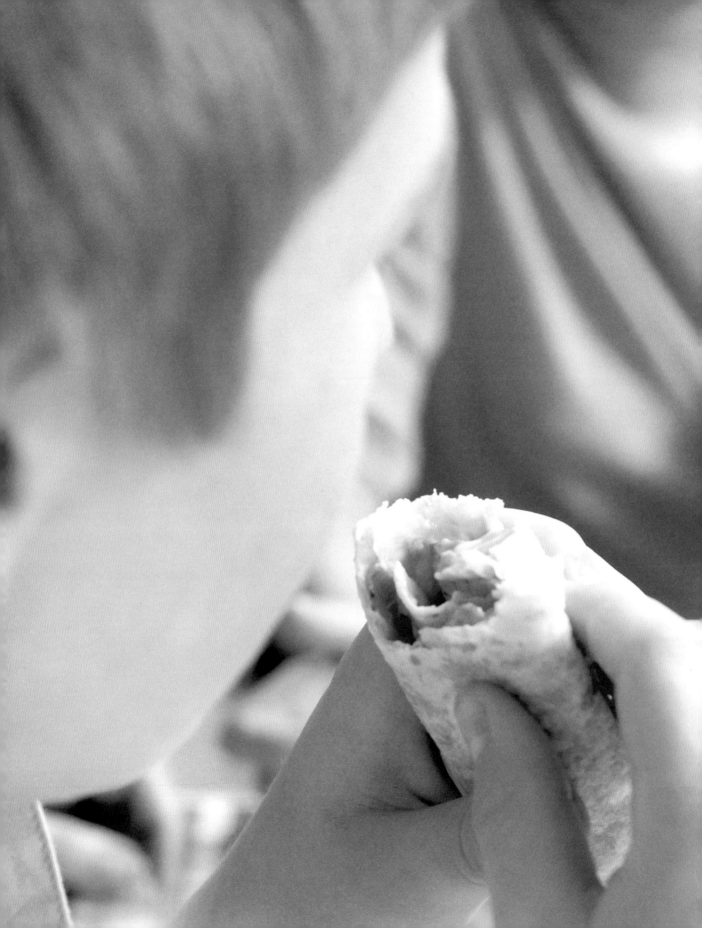

Reuben's Deli Wraps

These wraps make a great nutritious lunch for kids and adults. Parents seem to love their fresh-from-the-deli taste, and kids feel very grown-up eating them. Serve with a baked potato for a meal, or on their own as a snack. This recipe is slightly adapted from one used by chef friend Brent Castle.

Serves 4		Serves 96
450g (1lb)	chicken breast	5.4kg (12lb)
	olive oil	
225g (8oz)	iceberg lettuce	2.7kg (6lb)
225g (8oz)	white cabbage	2.7kg (6lb)
225g (8oz)	carrots	2.7kg (6lb)
115g (4oz)	Cheddar cheese	1.3kg (3lb)
115g (4oz)	mayonnaise	1.3kg (3lb)
25g (1oz)	tomato ketchup	300g (10½oz)
4–8	tortilla wraps	96

Preheat the oven to 120°C/250°F/Gas ½.

Cut the chicken meat into fine slices and stir-fry in a little oil in a heavy-based pan until thoroughly cooked. (If making the larger quantity, bake the chicken strips in the oven preheated to 200°C/400°F/Gas 6 for 5–10 minutes until thoroughly cooked.)

Finely shred the lettuce and cabbage, and grate the carrots and cheese. Mix together the grated vegetables and cheese. Mix together the mayonnaise and tomato ketchup to make a sauce.

Brush the tortilla wraps with a little oil and put in the low preheated oven for 2 minutes to warm through.

Spoon a little of the sauce over the wraps, lay a slice or two of the chicken strips along the wrap and put a spoonful of the vegetable and cheese mix on top. Wrap up and serve.

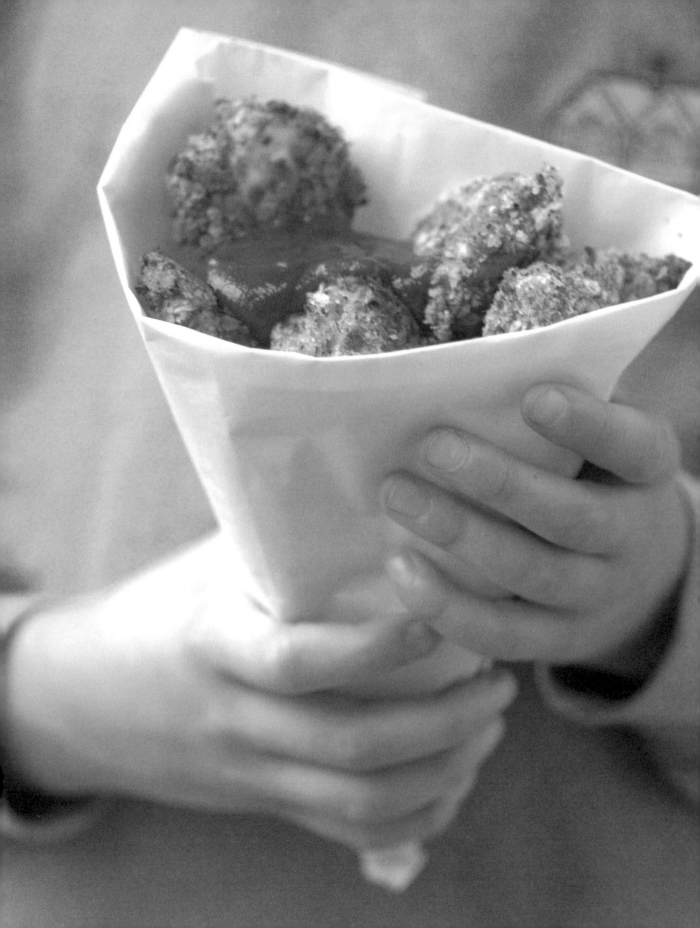

Real Chicken Nuggets

This is one of the simplest recipes in the book, and I'd much rather have the children eat these, made from local free-range or organic chicken, than any of the ingredients in the shop-bought chicken nugget. Get the children to help you make them – they love tossing the chicken in a bag of breadcrumbs. One adult portion will be roughly ten nuggets. Serve with some home-made tomato sauce or relish (see pages 124 and 208).

Serves 4		Serves 96
225g (8oz)	bread (brown or white)	2.7kg (6lb)
¹/₂ teaspoon	garlic powder	3 tablespoons
¹/₄ teaspoon	paprika	2 tablespoons
1	egg	12
125ml (4fl oz)	milk	1.5 litres (2¹/₂ pints)
900g (2lb)	diced chicken	10.8kg (24lb)

Preheat the oven to 200°C/400°F/Gas 6.

Slice the bread, then toast it until light brown. Break up into pieces, crusts and all, and reduce to fine crumbs in the food processor. Add the garlic powder and paprika, and whiz again. Place the breadcrumbs in a large plastic freezer bag or a deep tray.

Beat the egg in a large bowl with the milk, and add the chicken pieces, in batches if necessary. Transfer the chicken pieces to the bag or tray of breadcrumbs and toss to coat evenly.

Arrange the crumbed chicken on a lightly greased baking sheet, and bake in the preheated oven for 10 minutes until browned and crisp, and cooked through.

Lemon Chicken and Pea Risotto

I cannot do this recipe very often at the school – for so many children I need a very large pan. Use fresh peas when in season; cook them first in boiling water then drain. When serving, you could add some grated Parmesan or Cheddar, if you liked.

Serves 4		Serves 96
1	lemon	12
1	garlic clove	12
450g (1lb)	chicken strips	5.4kg (12lb)
1 tablespoon	olive oil	175ml (6fl oz)
550g (1¼lb)	risotto rice	6.75kg (15lb)
4	chicken stock cubes	36
1.7 litres (3 pints)	boiling water	20 litres (36 pints)
450g (1lb)	frozen peas	5.4kg (12lb)

Preheat the oven to 200°C/400°F/Gas 6.

Wash the lemon, and finely grate the zest off. Juice the lemon. Peel and crush the garlic.

Place the chicken strips in a deep tin. Pour the lemon juice and grated zest over and cook in the preheated oven for 15–20 minutes.

Meanwhile, heat the garlic and olive oil together in a large saucepan, add the rice and stir to coat the rice with the oil. Dissolve the stock cubes in the boiling water, and keep at a simmer in a pan on top of the stove, next to the risotto pan. Gradually add the stock to the rice, stirring, allowing each lot to be absorbed before adding the next. Add the frozen peas when you've used up about half of the stock.

When all the stock has been used up, add the chicken strips and stir thoroughly. Serve straightaway.

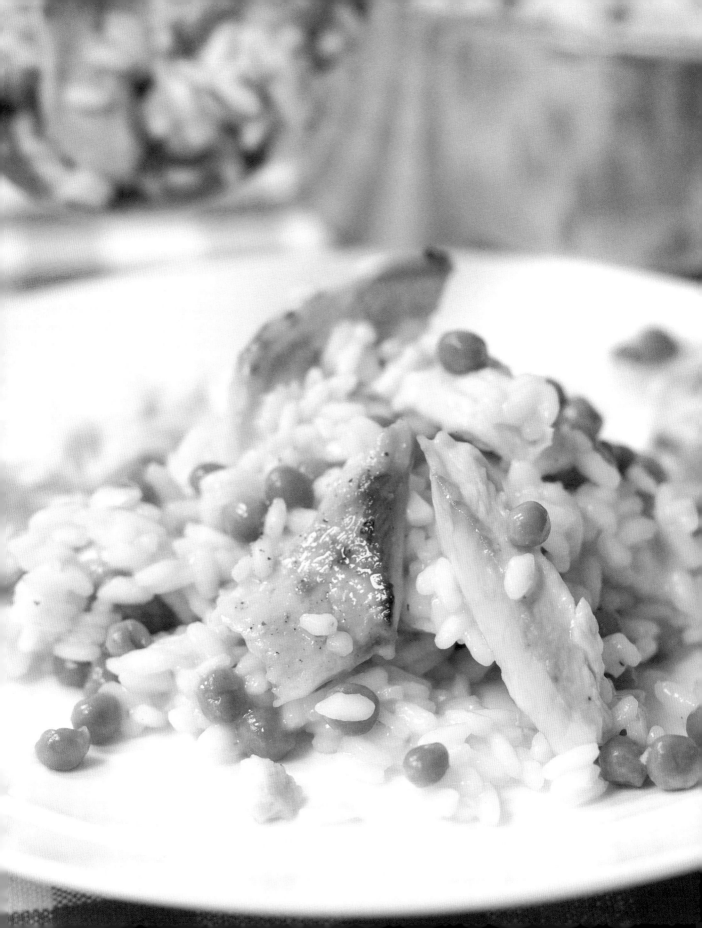

Turkey, Ham and Vegetable Pie

This is a filling dish, for the hungriest of appetites, and one in which you can use your imagination. Use any vegetable that is in season, and the pie will be different every time you make it. Hopefully your children will be eating different vegetables without knowing – try tiny broccoli florets, carrots, peas, cauliflower or courgettes, to name but a few.

Serves 4		Serves 96
	Pastry	
225g (8oz)	plain flour	2.7kg (6lb)
55g (2oz)	margarine	675g (1½lb)
55g (2oz)	vegetable shortening	675g (1½lb)
25ml (1fl oz)	water	350ml (12fl oz)
	Filling	
225g (8oz)	onions	2.7kg (6lb)
225g (8oz)	fresh mixed vegetables	2.7kg (6lb)
450g (1lb)	diced turkey	5.4kg (12lb)
1 tablespoon	olive oil	175ml (6fl oz)
1 sprig	fresh rosemary	5 sprigs
225g (8oz)	cooked ham, diced	2.7kg (6lb)
	Sauce	
300ml (10fl oz)	turkey liquid (see method)	3.4 litres (6 pints)
300ml (10fl oz)	milk	3.4 litres (6 pints)
½	lemon	6
55g (2oz)	butter or margarine	675g (1½lb)
55g (2oz)	plain flour	675g (1½lb)

For the pastry, sift the flour into a bowl. Cut the fats into cubes, add to the flour, and rub in until the mixture resembles breadcrumbs. Add the water and mix with a knife until you have a dough. Wrap in clingfilm and put in the fridge.

Peel and chop the onions, and prepare the fresh mixed vegetables as appropriate.

Fry the turkey and onions in a little oil until coloured all over, but not brown, then add enough water to just cover the meat, along with the rosemary. Simmer until tender, add the mixed vegetables and ham and cook for a further 5–10 minutes, until the vegetables are just cooked. Drain, reserving the stock. Mix the stock with the milk and lemon juice for the sauce.

Meanwhile, preheat the oven to 190°C/375°F/Gas 5.

To make the sauce, melt the butter or margarine in a pan, then add the flour and cook over a gentle heat until the mixture turns sandy in colour and texture. Gradually add the reserved turkey stock and milk mixture, and cook until the mixture thickens. Mix with the turkey, ham and vegetables, and place in a suitable dish or tin.

Roll the pastry out to cover the dish or tin, brush with a little extra milk, and bake in the preheated oven until the pastry is golden brown, about 35–40 minutes.

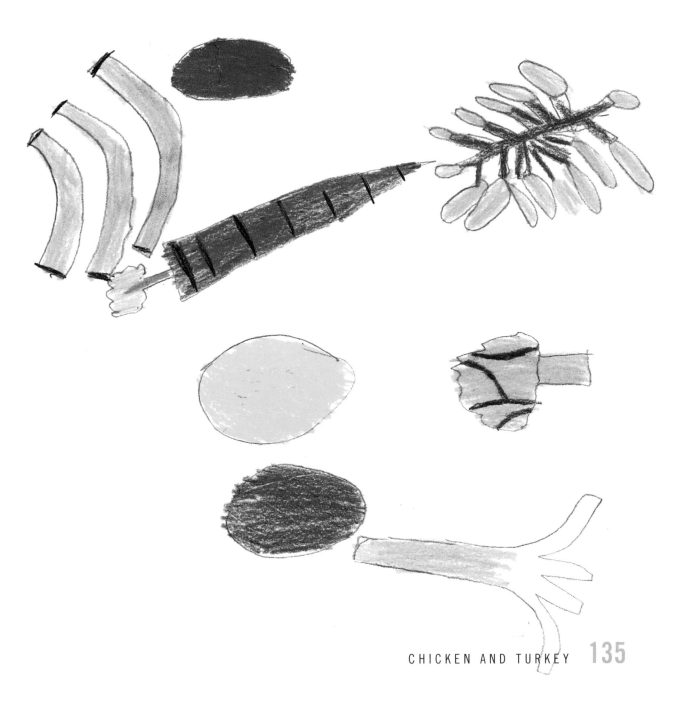

Roast Chicken

Of all the roast dinners we do at St Peter's this is the children's favourite, with roast lamb coming a close second. People say that children nowadays don't want to eat good food. Well, come to our school on a Wednesday, and you will see the children tucking into a roast dinner. In fact, the numbers go up all the time as more children want to stay, and the parents come as well. I use boned and rolled chicken breast in the school kitchen, as this gives me the minimum amount of waste, but at home you would use a whole chicken. We use fresh free-range chicken, which comes from a farm in Lincolnshire, or organic chicken, which comes from the Derbyshire Dales.

Serves 4		Serves 96
1.5kg (3lb)	chicken flavourings (see below)	10.8kg (24lb)

Preheat the oven to 190°C/375°F/Gas 5.

For the whole chicken, put in a roasting tray. Add flavourings to the body cavity if liked – ½ lemon, a few fresh herbs, a garlic clove or two. Put a little water in the bottom of the tray, and roast in the preheated oven, allowing 20 minutes per 450g (1lb), plus 20 minutes, or until the juices run clear when the thickest part of the thigh is pierced with a skewer.

For the rolled chicken, wrap the chicken roll in a piece of foil large enough to comfortably enclose it, not too tightly. Have the matt side inside. Don't add any flavourings. Simply roast, with a little water in the bottom of the tin, for the same calculated time.

Serve hot with gravy (see page 165), roast potatoes and seasonal vegetables.

> **"**The best thing about school dinners is Mrs Orrey, because she's nice to us. And I like having the old people to lunch.**"**
> LILY GILBERT, 7

Chicken, Ham and Egg Pie

This is a really tasty recipe, quick and old-fashioned, and can be served hot or cold. It's something I've introduced recently into the school menu.

Serves 4		Serves 96
2	eggs	24
225g (8oz)	cooked chicken meat	2.7kg (6lb)
225g (8oz)	cooked gammon or ham	2.7kg (6lb)
	Pastry	
225g (8oz)	plain flour	2.7kg (6lb)
55g (2oz)	margarine	675g (1½lb)
55g (2oz)	vegetable shortening	675g (1½lb)
25ml (1fl oz)	water	350ml (12fl oz)
	White sauce	
55g (2oz)	butter or margarine	675g (1½lb)
55g (2oz)	plain flour	675g (1½lb)
600ml (1 pint)	milk	6.8 litres (12 pints)
1 teaspoon	English mustard	55g (2oz)
1 teaspoon	finely grated lemon zest	55g (2oz)
3 tablespoons	chopped parsley	150g (5½oz)

For the pastry, sift the flour into a bowl. Cut the margarine and vegetable shortening into cubes, add to the flour, and rub in until the mixture resembles breadcrumbs. Add the water and mix with a knife until you have a dough. Wrap in clingfilm and put in the fridge.

Cook the eggs in boiling water for 8 minutes, then leave in cold water until cool. Shell and roughly chop. Cut the chicken and ham into chunky pieces.

To make the white sauce, melt the butter or margarine in a saucepan then add the flour and cook, stirring, until sandy in colour and texture. Add the milk, whisking all the time. When the sauce has thickened, add the mustard, lemon zest and parsley, and put to one side.

Preheat the oven to 180°C/350°F/Gas 4.

Take the pastry out of the fridge and divide into two pieces. On a floured board roll one piece out until big enough to line a 1.4 litre (2½ pint) pie dish. Trim off any excess.

Put the chicken, ham and hard-boiled egg into the pastry-lined dish, and pour over the white sauce. Roll out the remaining pastry to form a lid for the pie. Dampen the edges of this and the pastry in the dish, and place on top. Press the edges together. Brush the top with milk, and make a slit in the middle of the pastry to let the steam out. Bake in the preheated oven until golden brown, about 30–35 minutes.

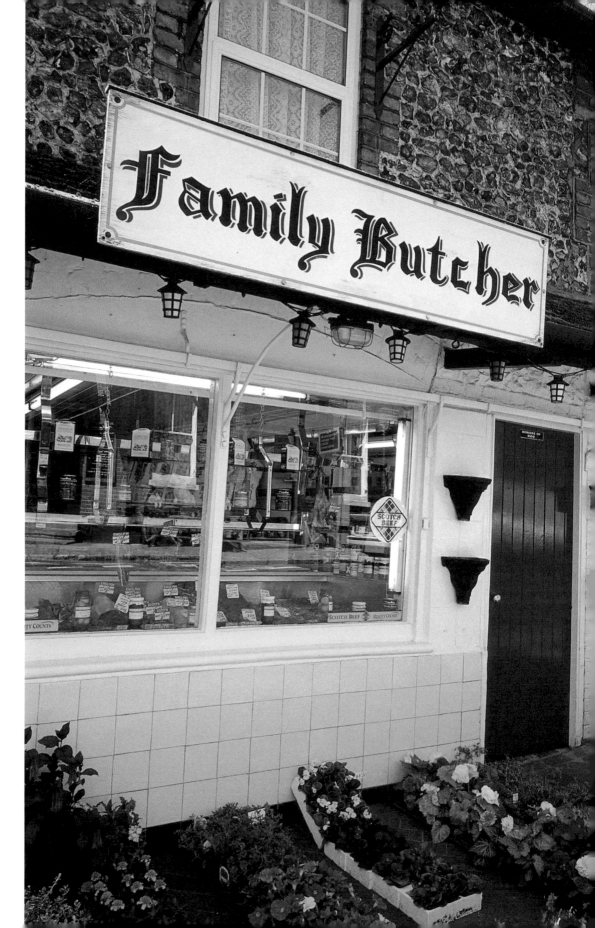

Pork, Beef and Lamb

Pasta, Peas and Bacon

This is so good that it was awarded five stars in the British Meat & Livestock Commission School Meals Catering Excellence Award, 2001. Serve with wholemeal bread rolls.

Serves 4		Serves 96
250g (9oz)	onions	1.3kg (3lb)
175g (6oz)	Cheddar cheese	2kg (4½lb)
85g (3oz)	margarine	1kg (2¼lb)
225g (8oz)	lean diced bacon	2.7kg (6lb)
175g (6oz)	frozen peas	2kg (4½lb)
225g (8oz)	pasta shapes	2.7kg (6lb)
	olive oil	
40ml (1½fl oz)	milk	500ml (18fl oz)

Preheat the oven to 180°C/350°F/Gas 4.

Peel and chop the onions, and grate the cheese. Melt the margarine in a saucepan, add the onion and fry until soft. Add the diced bacon, and continue to fry gently until the bacon is thoroughly cooked. Add the peas and continue cooking slowly over a low heat for about 5–6 minutes.

In a separate saucepan, cook the pasta in boiling water. When al dente, drain, rinse and sprinkle with a little olive oil to prevent sticking.

When the bacon mixture is cooked, add the pasta, milk and half or all the cheese, and stir gently to combine until the cheese has melted. You can serve this straightaway, or put into an ovenproof dish, sprinkle with the remaining cheese, and put into the preheated oven for approximately 10–15 minutes, or until bubbling.

❝ I'm proud that our food's coming from farmers nearby. It's silly that food goes all over the country before people eat it. ❞

MEGAN SWEET, 10

Sausage Casserole

This is always popular, and I like to serve it on a chilly winter's day. Baked beans can be used instead of the tomatoes (a version of Cowboy Casserole; see page 147), or you could have a mixture of baked beans and canned tomatoes.

Serves 4		Serves 96
16	thin sausages	192
115g (4oz)	onions	1.3kg (3lb)
	vegetable oil	
2 x 400g cans	chopped tomatoes	3 x A10 (2.6kg) cans
a pinch	dried mixed herbs	2 teaspoons
150ml (5fl oz)	water	1.7 litres (3 pints)

Preheat the oven to 200°C/400°F/Gas 6.

Cut the sausages into three pieces each, and peel and chop the onions. Put the sausage pieces and onions in a lightly oiled ovenproof dish, and bake in the preheated oven for 15–20 minutes.

Add the chopped tomatoes, herbs and water to the sausages, cover the dish and bake in the preheated oven for 45 minutes.

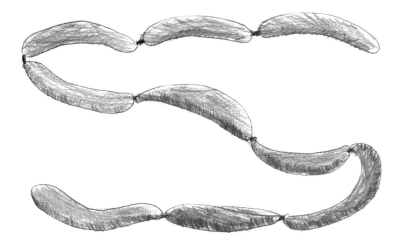

Barbecue Pork

This recipe introduces children to different tastes and textures. I make it here with pork, but you could use turkey instead. You could also use canned pineapple instead of peaches. It's good served with rice. In the spring, you could add spring onions, French beans or mangetouts.

Serves 4		Serves 96
225g (8oz)	onions	2kg (4¹/₂lb)
225g (8oz)	carrots	2kg (4¹/₂lb)
175g (6oz)	courgettes	2kg (4¹/₂lb)
1 x 400g can	peaches in juice	6 x 400g cans
2 tablespoons	olive oil	350ml (12fl oz)
450g (1lb)	diced pork	5.4kg (12lb)
	black pepper	
115g (4oz)	tomato purée	1.3kg (3lb)
40ml (1¹/₂fl oz)	vinegar	425ml (15fl oz)
¹/₂ tablespoon	caster sugar	200g (7oz)
¹/₂ teaspoon	ready-mixed mustard	25g (1oz)
¹/₂	lemon	6
400ml (14fl oz)	water and peach juice	4.8 litres (8 pints)
55g (2oz)	sultanas (optional)	675g (1¹/₂lb)

Preheat the oven to 180°C/350°F/Gas 4.

Peel and slice the onions. Peel and dice the carrots. Trim and dice the courgettes. Drain the peaches, keeping both peaches and juices. Heat half the olive oil in a pan, add the onions and carrots and allow them to soften over a medium heat for about 10 minutes. Transfer to a casserole. Season the meat with black pepper, add to the pan in batches, and fry in the remaining olive oil until sealed, a few minutes. Transfer to the casserole, then fry the next batch.

Mix the tomato purée, vinegar, sugar, mustard, lemon juice and the water and peach juices together in a bowl. Add to the meat and onions in the casserole along with the sultanas (if using). Cover and cook in the preheated oven until tender, about 30 minutes.

Cut the peaches into pieces, add to the meat, and return to the oven for a further 15 minutes.

Home-made Pork Balls with Spaghetti

We can't make enough of these! The kids love them and always ask for more.
Serve them with the tomato sauce on page 124.

Serves 4		Serves 96
450g (1lb)	spaghetti	*5.4kg (12lb)*
1 tablespoon	olive oil	*175ml (6fl oz)*
	fresh tomato sauce (see page 124)	
2 tablespoons	chopped oregano	*6 tablespoons*
Meatballs		
55g (2oz)	Cheddar cheese	*675g (1½lb)*
2	garlic cloves	*5*
450g (1lb)	minced pork	*5.4kg (12lb)*
150g (5½oz)	fresh white breadcrumbs	*1.8kg (4lb)*
1 tablespoon	chopped parsley	*6 tablespoons*
1 tablespoon	chopped sage	*6 tablespoons*
1	egg	*12*

Preheat the oven to 180°C/350°F/Gas 4.

For the meatballs, grate the Cheddar, and peel and crush the garlic.

Mix the pork mince, cheese, garlic, breadcrumbs, herbs and egg together with sufficient water to bind. Divide into about 16 balls and place in a well-greased ovenproof dish. Bake in the preheated oven for about 35–40 minutes, shaking the dish every now and again, until golden brown.

Meanwhile, cook the spaghetti in boiling water until al dente. Drain and sprinkle with a little olive oil to stop it sticking together. Warm the tomato sauce through. Pour the meatballs and sauce on top of the spaghetti, and sprinkle with the chopped oregano.

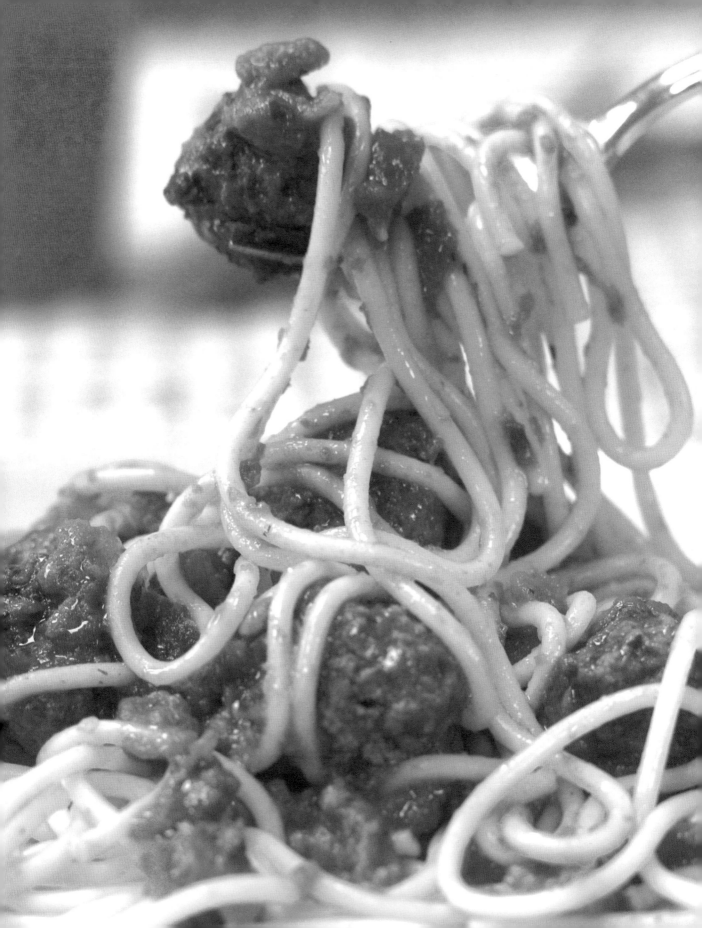

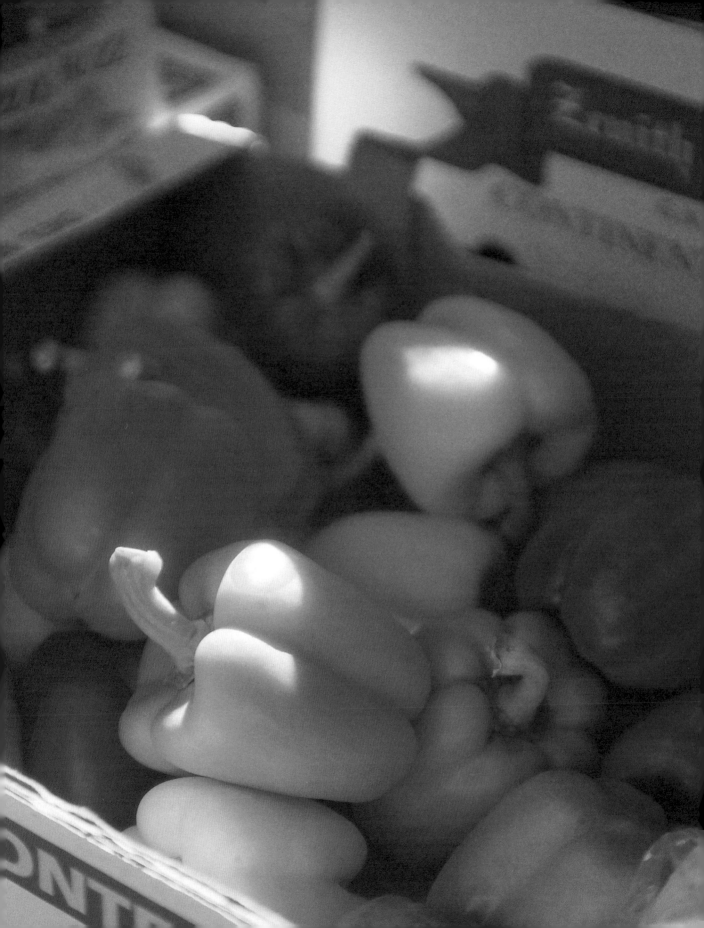

Sizzling Sausage

This is a great way for children to eat vegetables and rice

Serves 4		Serves 96
350g (12oz)	long-grain rice	4kg (9lb)
275g (10oz)	chipolata sausages	3kg (7lb)
1	red pepper	12
1	green pepper	12
175g (6oz)	onions	2kg (4½lb)
1 tablespoon	olive oil	175ml (6fl oz)
175g (6oz)	frozen sweetcorn	2kg (4½lb)
175g (6oz)	frozen peas	2kg (4½lb)

Preheat the oven to 180°C/350°F/Gas 4.

Place the rice in a sieve and rinse under cold running water. Bring a pan of water to the boil, add the rice, and return to the boil. Stir once then reduce the heat, cover and simmer for about 11 minutes or until tender. Drain in a sieve, rinse with boiling water, cover and keep warm.

Meanwhile, cut the sausages into three and put into an ovenproof dish. Cook in the preheated oven for 10–12 minutes or until golden brown.

Seed and finely dice the peppers. Peel and finely chop the onions. Heat the oil in a large frying pan and gently cook the pepper and onion until soft and lightly golden.

Meanwhile, bring a pan of water to the boil. Add the sweetcorn and peas, bring back to the boil, and cook for 2 minutes. Drain. Add to the peppers and onions.

Remove the sausages from the oven, drain off excess liquid and add the sausages to the pan. Stir in the cooked rice over a low heat until hot and sizzling. Serve immediately.

Pork and Apple Casserole

This recipe is really tasty made with free-range pork, but to push the boat out, ask your butcher if he can get you some Gloucester Old Spot pork. This is increasingly available, and is full of flavour. You could add also some beans or peas to the casserole at the same time as the apple. If you have a slow-cooker – a very economical piece of kitchen equipment – you could make this the night before, adding the apple when you get home from work.

Serves 4		Serves 96
675g (1½lb)	diced shoulder pork	8kg (18lb)
225g (8oz)	onions	2.7kg (6lb)
225g (8oz)	carrots	2.7kg (6lb)
225g (8oz)	cooking apples	2.7kg (6lb)
	lemon juice	
	olive oil	
a pinch	dried sage	2 teaspoons
½ level teaspoon	Marmite	25g (1oz)
600ml (1 pint)	hot water	6.8 litres (12 pints)
25g (1oz)	cornflour	350g (12oz)

Preheat the oven to 170°C/325°F/Gas 3.

Wash and pat the meat dry with kitchen paper. Peel and chop the onions and carrots. Core and peel the cooking apples; slice them and put in some water acidulated with lemon juice until ready to use.

Fry the meat and onions in batches in a little oil until browned on all sides, and put in a deep tin. Add the carrots and sage, and cover with a stock made with the Marmite and hot water. Cover, and bake in the preheated oven until the meat is tender, about 2–2½ hours. I like to slow-cook all my casseroles to bring out the flavour.

About 15 minutes before the end of cooking, blend the cornflour with a little water, and add to the stew to thicken, along with the drained apples. Stir in well, and continue cooking until the apple is tender.

Cowboy Casserole

This is very easy and children love it. If you buy good-quality sausages and bacon, less fat will come out of them. If you do see some fat, drain it off before adding the beans. Use low sugar and salt baked beans for this recipe, and serve with a jacket potato.

Serves 4		Serves 96
16	thin sausages	*192*
225g (8oz)	diced lean bacon	*2.7kg (6lb)*
2 x 400g cans	baked beans	*3 x A10 (2.6kg) cans*

Preheat the oven to 200°C/400°F/Gas 6.

Cut the sausages into small pieces. Put these into a deep tin with the bacon, and bake in the preheated oven for 10–15 minutes until just golden brown.

Add the beans to the sausage and bacon, cover with foil or a lid, and cook for a further 25–30 minutes. Serve hot.

❝ Me and my friends really like football, but we're only allowed to play if we've eaten everything on our plates. That's not hard – it's always delicious. I bet David Beckham used to eat his school dinners. ❞

CONNOR COFFEY, 8

Toad in the Hole

The children always ask why this dish is called by this name. I don't know the answer. Do you?

Serves 4		Serves 96
2 tablespoons	olive oil	*300ml (10fl oz)*
8	thick sausages	*96*
	Yorkshire pudding	
115g (4oz)	plain flour	*1.3kg (3lb)*
a pinch	black pepper	*1/2 teaspoon*
1	egg	*12*
300ml (10fl oz)	milk	*3.4 litres (6 pints)*

To start the Yorkshire, sift the flour and pepper into a bowl and make a well in the centre. Beat the egg and add to the flour, along with half the milk. Beat well until the batter is smooth, then add the remaining milk. Put to one side while the oven heats up to 220°C/425°F/Gas 7.

Heat the oil in a small roasting tin on top of the stove, and add the sausages. Bake in the preheated oven for about 10 minutes, until just browned. Reduce the oven temperature to 200°C/400°F/Gas 6.

Remove the sausages from the oven and quickly pour the batter into the tin around the sausages. Put back into the oven immediately, and bake until risen and golden brown, a further 30–35 minutes.

**" My favourite dinner's the roast.
I like the fact that the meat comes from nearby,
so it's better for the planet. "**
JAKE GARLAND, 9

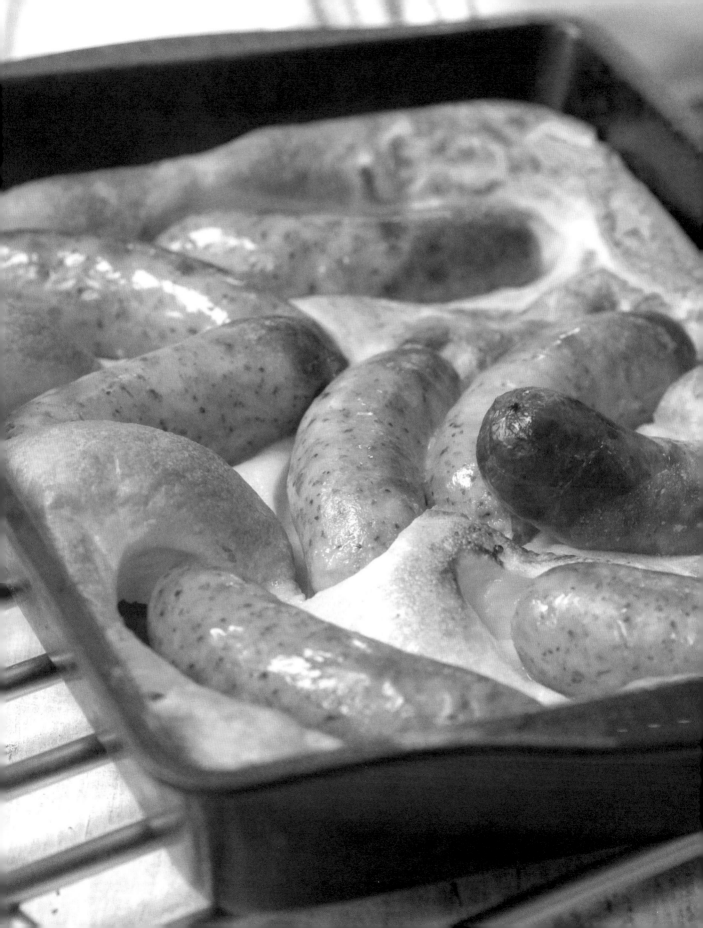

Pancake Pizza

Brent Castle, a chef who has his own pub/restaurant, first cooked this at St Peter's when he came for the day to promote British beef with the Meat & Livestock Commission. It is a regular on my menu now.

Serves 4		Serves 96
225g (8oz)	onions	2.7kg (6lb)
225g (8oz)	courgettes	2.7kg (6lb)
225g (8oz)	peppers (green or red)	2.7kg (6lb)
8	tomatoes	48
1 tablespoon	olive oil	175ml (6fl oz)
450g (1lb)	minced beef	5.4kg (12lb)
1 tablespoon	plain flour	175g (6oz)
1 teaspoon	paprika	5 teaspoons
1	beef stock cube	2
175ml (6fl oz)	boiling water	1.7 litres (3 pints)
1 x 400g jar	tomato passata	12 x 400g cans
8	tortilla wraps	96
	Cheese sauce	
225g (8oz)	Cheddar cheese	2.7kg (6lb)
25g (1oz)	butter or margarine	350g (12oz)
25g (1oz)	plain flour	350g (12oz)
600ml (1 pint)	milk	6.8 litres (12 pints)

Peel and chop the onions. Trim and chop the courgettes. Halve the peppers and remove the seeds, then chop the flesh. Slice the tomatoes. Grate the cheese for the sauce.

Heat some of the oil in a large pan, add the mince and onion, and fry gently to brown. Remove from the pan and drain any excess fat off. Return the pan to the stove, add a little more oil, and sauté the courgettes and peppers until they are golden brown.

Return the minced beef to the pan with the vegetables, sprinkle in the flour and paprika, and stir to combine. Mix the beef stock cube and boiling water, and add this and the tomato passata to the beef. Simmer until the vegetables are tender and the sauce is a thick moist consistency, about 25–30 minutes.

To make the cheese sauce, melt the butter or margarine in a saucepan, add the flour and cook until sandy in colour and texture. Add the milk all at once, stirring all the time, and continue to simmer and stir until thickened. Remove from the heat and add half the grated cheese.

Preheat the oven to 200°C/400°F/Gas 6.

To make up the pancake pizzas, put the tortillas in an oiled dish, cover with foil, and warm through in the preheated oven for 2–5 minutes. Fill each tortilla with the meat mixture and fold into a roll. Arrange side by side in a dish and top with the cheese sauce. Lay tomato slices on each portion, and sprinkle with the remaining grated cheese. Bake in the preheated oven until browned on top, about 15 minutes.

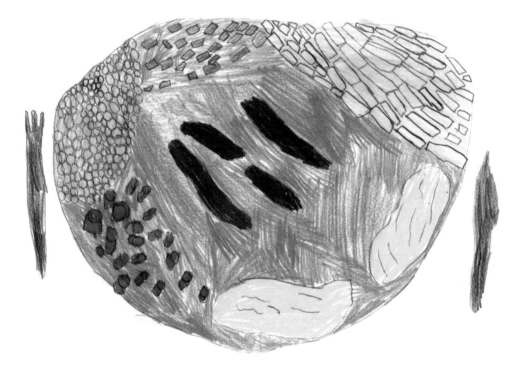

Beef and Potato Pie

This started off life as a beef, carrot and potato pie, but you can add any root vegetable since they are so full of flavour and have good texture. As well as those I've suggested here, celeriac would be good.

Serves 4		Serves 96
	Pastry	
225g (8oz)	plain flour	2.7kg (6lb)
55g (2oz)	margarine	675g (1¹/₂lb)
55g (2oz)	vegetable shortening	675g (1¹/₂lb)
25ml (1fl oz)	water	350ml (12fl oz)
	Filling	
175g (6oz)	carrots and parsnips	1.8kg (4lb)
175g (6oz)	onions and turnips	1.8kg (4lb)
1 tablespoon	olive oil	175ml (6fl oz)
600g (1lb 5oz)	diced beef	6.7kg (15lb)
25g (1oz)	plain flour	350g (12oz)
600ml (1 pint)	water	7.2 litres (12¹/₂ pints)
¹/₂ level teaspoon	Marmite	55g (2oz)
450g (1lb)	potatoes	5.4kg (12lb)

Preheat the oven to 150°C/300°F/Gas 2.

For the beef filling, peel the root vegetables, then wash and dice. Peel and slice the onions.

Heat the oil in a large flameproof casserole, and fry the meat and onions until the meat is sealed. Mix the flour with a little of the water until smooth, then add to the casserole along with the rest of the water, Marmite and vegetables (apart from the potatoes). Put the lid on, and cook in the preheated oven until the meat is tender, about 2 hours.

Meanwhile, make the pastry. Sift the flour into a large bowl. Cut the margarine and vegetable shortening into cubes, add to the flour, and rub in until the mixture resembles breadcrumbs. Add the water and mix with a knife until it looks like a ball. Wrap in clingfilm and chill for about half an hour.

Turn the oven up to 220°C/425°F/Gas 7.

Peel and cut the potatoes into cubes. Bring to the boil in a separate pan of water, and cook until still firm. Drain. Mix with the warm beef stew.

Roll out the pastry to fit the top of the casserole, then put in place, and neaten the edges. Bake in the preheated oven for 30–40 minutes, or until the pastry is golden.

Goulash

This is a good winter filler, and you can choose which meat to use – lamb, pork or beef. I know it should be beef, but I am feeding children, and they can get bored with eating the same meat all the time. Serve with vegetables and crusty bread rolls.

Serves 4		Serves 96
450g (1lb)	diced meat	5.4kg (12lb)
175g (6oz)	onions	1.8kg (4lb)
450g (1lb)	potatoes	5.4kg (12lb)
1 tablespoon	olive oil	175ml (6fl oz)
70g (2½oz)	tomato purée	800g (1¾lb)
½ level teaspoon	paprika	2 tablespoons
600ml (1 pint)	water	6.8 litres (12 pints)
½ level teaspoon	Marmite	55g (2oz)
25g (1oz)	plain flour	350g (12oz)

Wash and drain the meat in a colander, then pat dry with kitchen paper. Peel and finely chop the onions. Peel and cut the potatoes into small cubes (store in water until needed).

Heat the oil in a large casserole, and fry the onion until soft, about 5 minutes. Remove the onion with a slotted spoon and set aside. Add half the quantity of meat to the pan and fry over a high heat until lightly golden on each side. Remove and set aside and repeat with the remaining meat.

Return the onions and meat to the casserole with the tomato purée and paprika, and cook for 2–3 minutes. Add the drained diced potatoes, cover with the water and stir in the Marmite. Bring to the boil, reduce the heat, cover and simmer gently for about 1 hour or until the meat is tender.

Just before serving, blend the flour with a little cold water, and add to the meat through a sieve, stirring carefully until thickened.

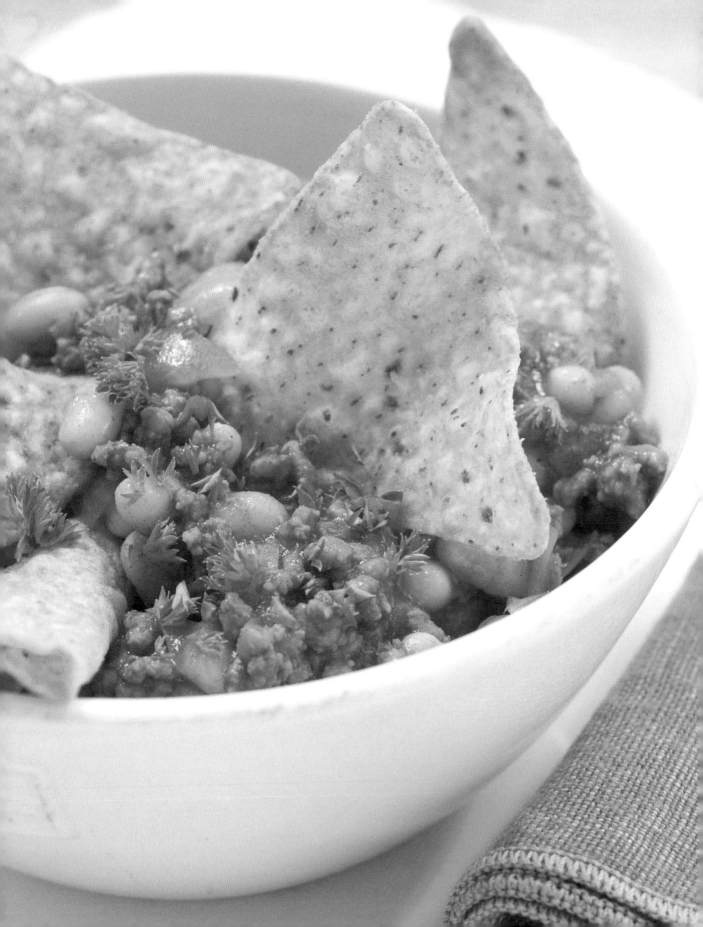

Chilli con Carne

My beef comes from a farm shop, which is five miles from the school. The beef is hung for a minimum of three weeks. It's important to have a good relationship with your butcher – his or her knowledge can be so useful. Instead of boiled rice, you could also serve this with tortilla chips. Use low sugar and salt baked beans.

Serves 4		Serves 96
175g (6oz)	onions	*1.6kg (3¾lb)*
1 tablespoon	olive oil	*175ml (6fl oz)*
450g (1lb)	minced beef	*5.4kg (12lb)*
½ teaspoon	chilli powder	*25g (1oz)*
a pinch	dried oregano	*2 teaspoons*
115g (4oz)	tomato purée	*1.3kg (3lb)*
1 x 400g can	baked beans	*6 x 800g cans*
175g (6oz)	patna rice	*2kg (4½lb)*

Peel and chop the onions. Heat the olive oil in a saucepan and fry the onion and mince together until the meat has browned and the onion softened. Add the chilli powder and oregano and cook for 1–2 minutes. Just cover with water, put the lid on and cook gently for 25 minutes.

Add the tomato purée and baked beans, and cook for a further 25–30 minutes, removing the lid and turning the heat up slightly for the last 5 minutes.

Meanwhile, cook the rice in boiling water until tender, about 15–20 minutes. Strain in a colander, rinse with boiling water, and drain well again.

Put the chilli into a bowl and serve with boiled rice.

Lamb Lasagne

I like to serve this popular dish with broccoli and a bread roll. If you want to use the lasagne that needs to be pre-cooked, simply drop into boiling water and cook for 3 minutes for fresh, about 8 for dried. A little nutmeg added to the cheese sauce is nice.

Serves 4		Serves 96
175g (6oz)	onions	*2kg (4½lb)*
175g (6oz)	carrots	*2kg (4½lb)*
450g (1lb)	minced lamb	*5.4kg (12lb)*
600ml (1 pint)	water	*5.4 litres (9 pints)*
115g (4oz)	tomato purée	*1.3kg (3lb)*
1 teaspoon	dried mixed herbs	*3 tablespoons*
225g (8oz)	pre-cooked lasagne	*2.7kg (6lb)*
	Cheese sauce	
225g (8oz)	Cheddar cheese	*2.7kg (6lb)*
25g (1oz)	butter or margarine	*500g (18oz)*
25g (1oz)	plain flour	*500g (18oz)*
600ml (1 pint)	milk	*5 litres (9 pints)*
1 teaspoon	wholegrain mustard	*3 teaspoons*

Preheat the oven to 200°C/400°F/Gas 6.

Peel and finely dice the onions. Scrub new carrots, peel old ones, then dice. Grate the cheese finely for the cheese sauce.

Dry-fry the meat until brown in a large frying pan, drain with a slotted spoon and transfer to a saucepan. In the same pan, cook the onion in the lamb fat until soft, about 3–5 minutes. Just cover the meat in the saucepan with water, then add the onion, carrot, tomato purée and dried herbs. Cover and cook until tender, about 30 minutes, then remove the lid, increase the heat, and bubble for a further 2–3 minutes to reduce if necessary.

To make the cheese sauce, melt the butter or margarine in a saucepan then add the flour, and cook, stirring, until sandy in texture and colour. Add the milk in one go and whisk vigorously so that no lumps develop. Cook for about 5 minutes. Add the mustard and nearly all the cheese, reserving a little for the top, and allow to melt. If too thick, add a little more milk.

Put half the lasagne in the base of the tin, and cover with half the meat sauce. Arrange a layer of the remaining lasagne over the meat, and then the remaining meat on top. Pour the cheese sauce over this, and sprinkle with the reserved cheese. Put into the preheated oven and bake until the pasta is tender and the top is brown, about 30–35 minutes.

Spaghetti Bolognaise

This is a great favourite with the children of St Peter's. Omit the mushrooms if your children don't like them. Two of my boys, Gareth and Jonathan, don't like them – in fact, mushrooms are the only thing they don't like to eat …

Serves 4		Serves 96
225g (8oz)	onions	2kg (4½lb)
225g (8oz)	carrots	2kg (4½lb)
225g (8oz)	red peppers	2kg (4½lb)
225g (8oz)	green peppers	2kg (4½lb)
175g (6oz)	mushrooms	450g (1lb)
175g (6oz)	Cheddar cheese	2kg (4½lb)
450g (1lb)	minced lamb	5.4kg (12lb)
600ml (1 pint)	water	6.8 litres (12 pints)
115g (4oz)	tomato purée	1.3kg (3lb)
1 teaspoon	dried mixed herbs	3 tablespoons
450g (1lb)	spaghetti	5.4kg (12lb)

Peel and finely chop the onions and carrots. Halve the peppers, remove the seeds, and cut the flesh into cubes. Trim the mushrooms and slice. Grate the cheese.

Dry-fry the mince in a saucepan until brown. Add the onion and carrot, the water and tomato purée, and simmer until the meat is almost cooked, about 20–30 minutes. Add the peppers, mushrooms and dried herbs.

Meanwhile, break the spaghetti into short lengths and cook in boiling water until al dente, about 15 minutes. (In the school kitchen, we then add the small pieces of spaghetti to the meat mixture, because when you are cooking for large numbers the cooked spaghetti can go sticky. This way we find the children can manage to eat it better.)

Arrange the sauce and spaghetti in dishes. Sprinkle with grated cheese, and serve immediately.

❝My favourite meal is the spaghetti Bolognese, but I like all of them.❞
CHARLOTTE HERMAN, 11

Moussaka

This recipe is very quick and easy to do, but the kids will think you have spent ages cooking.

Serves 4		Serves 96
225g (8oz)	onions	2.7kg (6lb)
1 tablespoon	olive oil	175ml (6fl oz)
450g (1lb)	minced lamb	5.4kg (12lb)
1 x 400g can	chopped tomatoes	2 x A10 (2.6kg) cans
675g (1½lb)	potatoes	6.75kg (15lb)
	Cheese sauce	
115g (4oz)	Cheddar cheese	1.3kg (3lb)
25g (1oz)	butter or margarine	350g (12oz)
25g (1oz)	plain flour	350g (12oz)
300ml (½pint)	milk	3.4 litres (6 pints)

Preheat the oven to 200°C/400°F/Gas 6.

Peel and finely chop the onions. Heat the oil in a large frying pan, add the onion and cook for 5 minutes or until soft. Add the lamb mince and cook, stirring, for another 4–5 minutes. Add the tomatoes and continue to cook for about 20–25 minutes.

Meanwhile, grate the cheese for the sauce and put aside. Peel and cut the potatoes in half. Put them into a large pan of water, bring up to the boil and simmer for about 15 minutes until they are just cooked. Drain and allow to cool a little, then cut into thick slices.

In a large shallow ovenproof dish, layer the meat with the potato slices, finishing with a neat layer of potato slices.

To make the cheese sauce, melt the butter or margarine in a saucepan, add the flour, and cook until sandy in colour and texture. Gradually stir in the milk to form a thick, smooth paste, and cook, stirring continuously, for 4–5 minutes. Add two-thirds of the cheese.

Pour the sauce over the potatoes and sprinkle with the reserved grated cheese. Place in the preheated oven to cook for about 25–30 minutes, or until golden and bubbling.

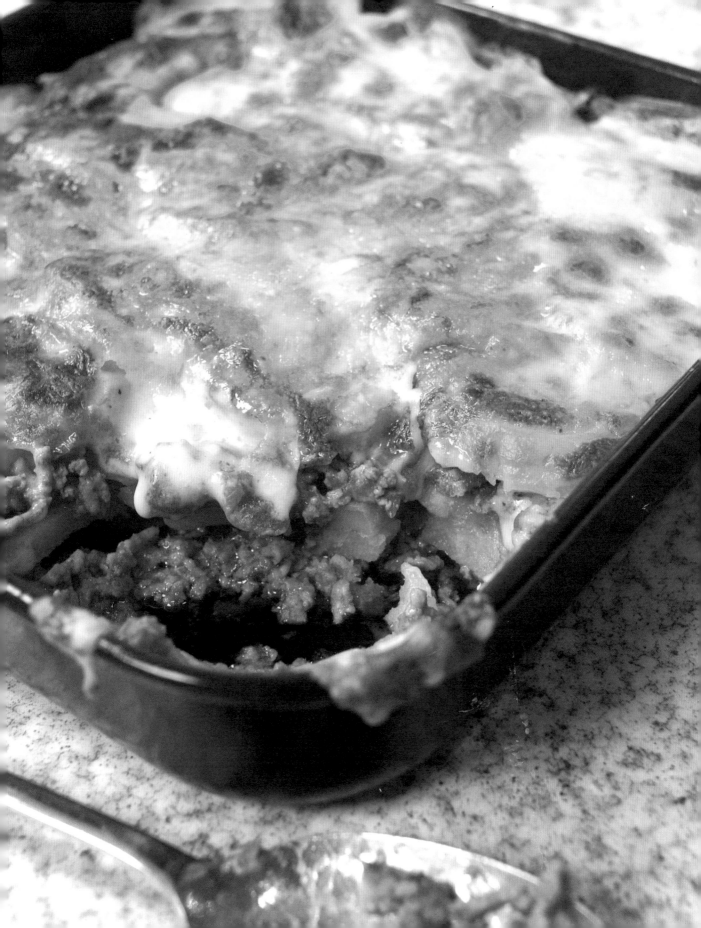

Lamb Cobbler

This is a hearty meal and you don't really need to serve potatoes, just some good vegetables that are in season.

Serves 4		Serves 96
225g (8oz)	onions	1.8kg (4lb)
225g (8oz)	carrots	2.7kg (6lb)
175g (6oz)	mushrooms	900g (2lb)
450g (1lb)	minced lamb	5.4kg (12lb)
½ level teaspoon	Marmite	55g (2oz)
25g (1oz)	plain flour	350g (12oz)
	Cobbler dough	
225g (8oz)	plain flour	2.7kg (6lb)
15g (½oz)	baking powder	175g (6oz)
55g (2oz)	butter or margarine	675g (1½lb)
150ml (5fl oz)	water	1.7 litres (3 pints)

Peel and dice the onions and carrots. Trim and slice the mushrooms.

Dry-fry the mince in a large saucepan until brown. Add the onion and carrot, and just enough water to cover. Mix the Marmite with a little hot water and add to the meat and vegetables. Simmer until almost cooked, about 25–35 minutes. Add the mushrooms and cook for a further 5–10 minutes. Preheat the oven to 200°C/400°F/Gas 6.

Strain the meat and vegetables into a deep ovenproof casserole, reserving the liquid in a small pan. Add a little water to the flour to make a smooth paste, then pour through a sieve into the reserved liquid. (I have a small stainless-steel sieve which is great for this job.) Stir over a gentle heat until thickened and cooked through, about 4–5 minutes. Pour over the meat and vegetables.

For the cobbler, sift the flour and baking powder into a bowl. Cut the butter or margarine into cubes, add it to the flour and rub it in until the texture is like breadcrumbs, then bring together into a dough with the water.

Roll the dough out and, using a 5cm (2in) plain cutter, cut out eight rounds. Place these on top of the meat, and bake in the preheated oven for 30–35 minutes until the cobbler is well risen.

Shepherd's Pie

A dish where you can hide the vegetables. Make sure you cut them very small. When I am asking the children which choice they would like, I call this one 'sheepdog pie', which always makes the little ones smile. This can be made in advance and frozen. To cook, defrost then bake according to the instructions in the recipe.

Serves 4		Serves 96
225g (8oz)	onions	*2kg (4¹/₂lb)*
225g (8oz)	carrots	*2kg (4¹/₂lb)*
¹/₂	red pepper	*4*
¹/₂	green pepper	*4*
1 tablespoon	olive oil	*175ml (6fl oz)*
450g (1lb)	minced lamb	*5.4kg (12lb)*
250ml (9fl oz)	water	*3 litres (5¹/₄ pints)*
1 level teaspoon	Marmite	*55g (2oz)*
25g (1oz)	plain flour	*350g (12oz)*
25g (1oz)	butter or margarine	*300g (10¹/₂oz)*
	Mashed potato	
900g (2lb)	potatoes	*10.8kg (24lb)*
50ml (2fl oz)	warm milk	*600ml (1 pint)*
25g (1oz)	butter or margarine	*300g (10¹/₂oz)*

Peel and chop the onions and carrots. Halve and seed the peppers, then chop.

Heat the oil in a large frying pan and cook the meat, onion, carrot and pepper until golden brown, about 10 minutes. Stir in the water with the Marmite. Simmer for a further 30–35 minutes.

Meanwhile, peel the potatoes and cut them into large chunks. Cook the potatoes in a pan of water until tender, about 20–25 minutes. Drain well and return to the pan. Mash the potatoes, then add the warm milk and the butter or margarine, and beat until fluffy and smooth.

Preheat the oven to 180°C/350°F/Gas 4.

Put the flour in a small bowl and add a little hot lamb liquid. Stir until you have a smooth paste, then pass through a sieve into the mince, stirring all the time. The mixture should be quite thick. Spoon the meat into a dish and top with the fluffy mashed potato. Dot the top with the remaining butter or margarine. Bake in the preheated oven for 25–30 minutes until golden brown and bubbling.

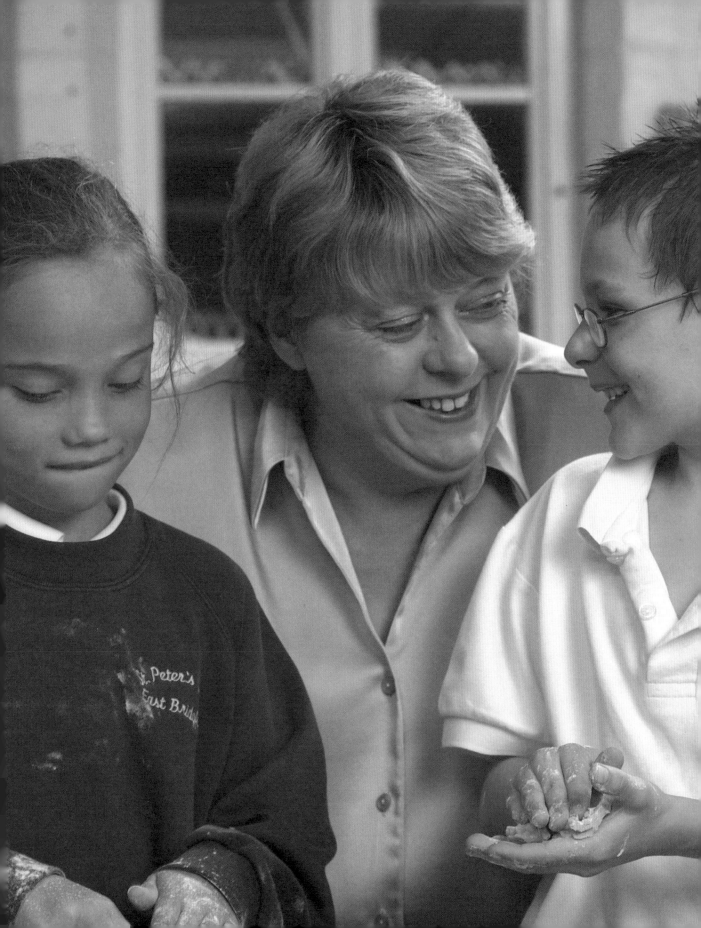

Lamb Casserole with Dumplings

The first time I made this, some of the children asked, 'What are those things in the stew?' I asked them to try the dumplings even if they only ate half, and most of them now love them, especially on a cold winter's day. Of course, you can omit the dumplings if you want a lighter dish. The longer you cook this at home, the better it tastes.

Serves 4		Serves 96
225g (8oz)	carrots	*2.7kg (6lb)*
225g (8oz)	onions	*1.8kg (4lb)*
350g (12oz)	potatoes	*4kg (9lb)*
115g (4oz)	button mushrooms	*1.3kg (3lb)*
450g (1lb)	diced lamb	*5.4kg (12lb)*
1 tablespoon	olive oil	*175ml (6fl oz)*
½ level teaspoon	Marmite	*55g (2oz)*
600ml (1 pint)	water	*6.8 litres (12 pints)*
25g (1oz)	plain flour	*350g (12oz)*
225g (8oz)	frozen peas	*2.7kg (6lb)*
	Dumplings	
225g (8oz)	plain flour	*2.7kg (6lb)*
15g (½oz)	baking powder	*175g (6oz)*
55g (2oz)	butter or margarine	*675g (1½lb)*
150ml (5fl oz)	water	*1.7 litres (3 pints)*

Preheat the oven to 180°C/350°F/Gas 4.

Peel and slice the carrots and dice the onions. Peel and dice the potatoes (and put in water). Quarter the mushrooms.

Brown half the meat in a saucepan in half of the oil, then transfer, using a slotted spoon, to a deep, lidded baking dish. Do the same with the remaining meat and oil. Add the carrots, onions, mushrooms, Marmite and water to the meat. Mix, cover and cook in the preheated oven for 1½–2 hours. The meat should be really tender.

Meanwhile, make the dumplings. Sift the flour and baking powder into a large bowl, add the butter or margarine cut into cubes, and rub into the flour until the mixture resembles breadcrumbs. Add the water and quickly mix well to form a soft dough. Turn the dough on to a floured work surface and cut into eight pieces. Lightly shape to form balls.

Remove the stew from the oven. Dissolve the flour in a little of the lamb juices, and return to the stew through a sieve. Mix in the peas and potato, then top with the dumplings, replace the lid and return to the oven for a further 40–45 minutes, turning the dumplings over halfway through if you like.

Remove from the oven, take the lid off, and watch the children's faces!

Roast Lamb

Roast lamb is the children's second favourite (next to roast chicken). The lamb we use at St Peter's comes from Gonalston Farm shop. The owners, Georgina and Ross Mason, are farmers as well. Georgina and I have a good relationship, and have become friends, both believing in what the other is trying to achieve. Arnold, the head butcher at the farm shop, also knows what I require for the children, and I only have to ask him for the cuts we require and it will be ready. Well done, Arnie, and thank you for putting up with me! At St Peter's we have a lot of visitors to the school, to see how we work, and I take them to the farm shop so they can see for themselves where and what we buy.

We use boned and rolled leg of lamb, partly because there is very little waste, and also because of time, as this cut does not require long slow cooking. I don't do anything fancy with a roast – I believe good meat needs nothing doing to it. And because I am feeding children, all my meat is well done.

Serves 4		Serves 96
1.3kg (3lb)	boned and rolled leg of lamb	10.8kg (24lb)
	black pepper	
1 tablespoon	olive oil	150ml (5fl oz)
1 bunch	fresh rosemary	5 bunches

Preheat the oven to 200°C/400°F/Gas 6.

Season the meat with lots of black pepper. Heat the oil in a roasting tray, and brown the meat on all sides. Scatter the rosemary across the bottom of the tray, lay the meat on top, and roast in the preheated oven for 20 minutes per 450g (1lb) plus 20 minutes, basting every now and again.

Leave to rest for about 15 minutes after removing from the oven. Serve with roast potatoes, broccoli, carrots or roasted cherry tomatoes (see page 193), plus gravy and mint sauce.

Meat Gravy

This gravy can go with any roast meat, if you use the relevant juices from the roasting tray and the relevant stock cube. The secret of good gravy, as we make it in the school kitchen, is to cook it for a good half an hour and not hurry it.

Serves 4		Serves 96
85g (3oz)	onions	*4 large*
25g (1oz)	butter or margarine	*350g (12oz)*
25g (1oz)	plain flour	*350g (12oz)*
750ml (26fl oz)	water	*6.8 litres (12 pints)*
1 teaspoon	Marmite	*1 tablespoon*
½	stock cube	*6*

Peel and slice the onions. Cook the onion in the butter or margarine until soft, then stir in the flour. Cook to brown the flour a little. Add the water, Marmite and stock cube – and fat-free juices from the roast – and stir well to avoid lumps. Bring to the boil, then reduce the heat to very low, and cook gently, covered, for about half an hour.

Strain the onions out, and serve the gravy hot.

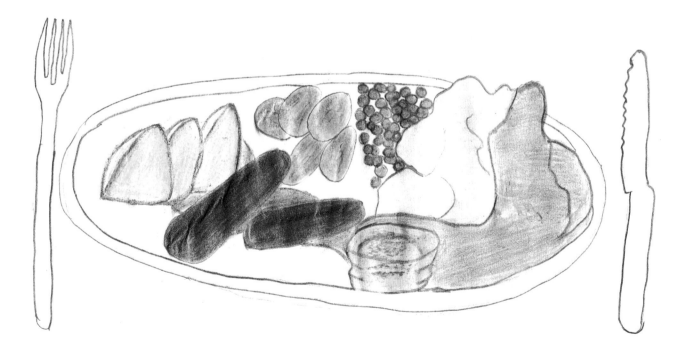

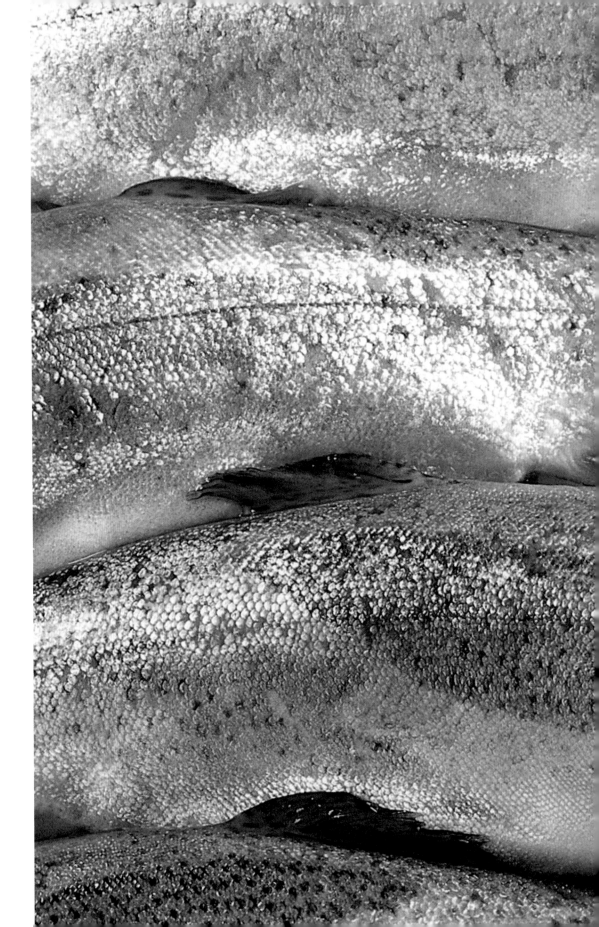

Fish

Fish Crumble Pie

Children love peas, and mixed with good fresh fish – such as skinless coley, cod or haddock – and topped with crisp breadcrumbs, they make a very good and colourful lunch dish. Use frozen peas. Mostly from nearby Lincolnshire, they are frozen immediately they are picked, so in fact can be fresher and richer in nutrients than peas in the pod, which might take a week to reach the shops . . .

Serves 4		Serves 96
450g (1lb)	boned white fish	5.4kg (12lb)
300ml (10fl oz)	milk	3.4 litres (6 pints)
2	eggs	24
225g (8oz)	frozen peas	2.7kg (6lb)
25g (1oz)	butter or margarine	350g (12oz)
25g (1oz)	plain flour	350g (12oz)
175g (6oz)	fresh breadcrumbs	2kg (4½lb)

Preheat the oven to 200°C/400°F/Gas 6.

Place the fish in a saucepan with enough of the milk to cover, and poach gently for about 5–10 minutes. Strain off the milk, and reserve both milk and fish. Pick over the fish just to check there are no residual bones or skin. Break the fish into large chunks and put into a casserole.

Hard-boil the eggs, about 8–10 minutes, then cover with cold water. Shell and chop.

Bring some water to the boil in a saucepan, and add the peas. Cook until tender, about 5 minutes. Drain well, and add the peas and chopped hard-boiled egg to the fish in the casserole.

To make a white sauce, melt the butter or margarine in a saucepan, add the flour and cook, stirring, until sandy in texture and colour. Gradually add the reserved fishy milk and the rest of the milk, stirring continuously, until the sauce thickens. Pour the sauce over the fish mixture, and mix gently.

Sprinkle the breadcrumbs over the top of the mixture, and cook in the preheated oven until the topping is brown and everything is cooked through, about 25 minutes.

Tuna Puffs

If you're short on time, try these – the kids will love them. For even more speed, use vol-au-vent cases. Bake the cases for the required time (check the packet). Mix the flaked tuna and most of the cheese, spoon into the baked cases and sprinkle with the remaining cheese. Put into a hot oven (220°C/425°F/Gas 7) for about 5 minutes, or until the cheese has melted.

Serves 4		Serves 96
1 x 500g packet	frozen puff pastry	*12 x 500g packets*
2 x 185g cans	tuna in brine	*12 x 185g cans*
85g (3oz)	Cheddar cheese	*1kg (2¼lb)*
	milk	

Leave the pastry to thaw at room temperature. Preheat the oven to 200°C/400°F/Gas 6.

Roll out the pastry until it is very thin, about 3mm (⅛in) thick. Cut into 12cm (4½in) squares (you should make about 18).

Drain the tuna well, then flake into a bowl. Grate the cheese and mix in with the tuna. Put a little of the tuna mixture in the middle of each pastry square. Dampen the edges of the pastry squares with water – using a brush or your finger. Fold one corner of each pastry square over to form a triangle.

Place the triangles on an oiled baking sheet, brush with milk and bake in the preheated oven until brown, about 10 minutes. Make sure the underneath is cooked.

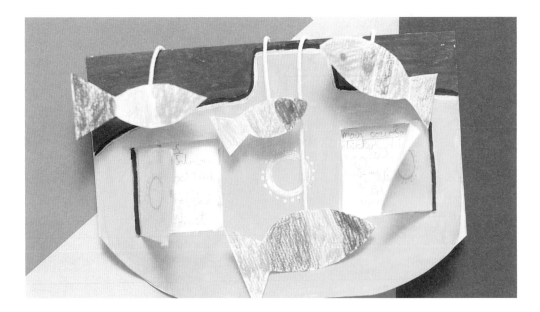

Fishy Pasta

I must admit that this one is seldom done in the kitchen – it's a treat for the children every now and again. The cream adds richness, but can be left out.

Serves 4		Serves 96
450g (1lb)	tricoloured pasta	5.4kg (12lb)
225g (8oz)	white fish fillets	2.7kg (6lb)
225g (8oz)	smoked haddock	2.7kg (6lb)
	milk	
	Sauce and topping	
1	leek	1.8–2.25kg (4–5lb)
175g (6oz)	Cheddar cheese	2kg (4½lb)
25g (1oz)	butter or margarine	350g (12oz)
25g (1oz)	plain flour	350g (12oz)
500ml (18fl oz)	milk	6 litres (10 pints)
50ml (2fl oz)	single cream	600ml (1 pint)
1 tablespoon	chopped parsley	6 tablespoons

Cook the pasta in boiling water until al dente, then drain well. Make sure the fish has no bones or skin. Clean and chop the leek for the sauce, and grate the cheese.

Poach the fish in a little milk to cover, for 5–10 minutes, then drain, reserving both. Break the fish into pieces.

For the sauce, melt the butter or margarine in a large pan. Add the leek and cook, stirring, for 1 minute. Add the flour and cook, stirring, for 1 minute. Gradually blend in the fishy milk and the rest of the milk, stirring constantly over a medium heat until the sauce boils and thickens. Reduce the heat and simmer for 3 minutes. Remove from the heat and stir in the grated Cheddar and cream. Add the fish and simmer for 1 minute. Remove from the heat.

Combine the fish mixture with the pasta and put into a warmed dish. Sprinkle with the parsley, and serve immediately.

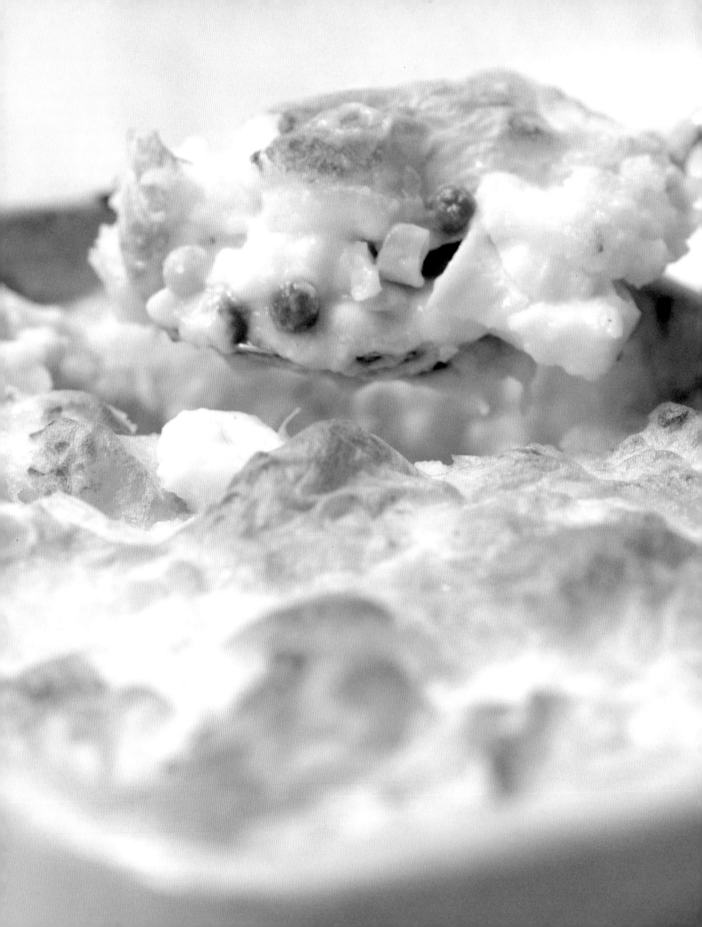

Fish Pie

Fresh fish is very hard for me to get hold of at school, as so many fishmongers have gone out of business. At the time of writing, I am talking to a man who comes round the village in a van delivering fish to the people of East Bridgford. You could make this pie with either peas or sweetcorn, or some of both, as here.

Serves 4		Serves 96
225g (8oz)	boned white fish	2.7kg (6lb)
225g (8oz)	smoked haddock	2.7kg (6lb)
	milk	
900g (2lb)	potatoes	10.8kg (24lb)
25g (1oz)	butter or margarine	300g (10½oz)
225g (8oz)	frozen sweetcorn	2.7kg (6lb)
85g (3oz)	frozen peas	1.3kg (3lb)
1 tablespoon	chopped parsley	6 tablespoons
	Cheese sauce	
175g (6oz)	Cheddar cheese	2kg (4½lb)
25g (1oz)	butter or margarine	350g (12oz)
25g (1oz)	plain flour	350g (12oz)
600ml (1 pint)	milk	6.8 litres (12 pints)
½ teaspoon	made mustard	2 teaspoons

Preheat the oven to 200°C/400°F/Gas 6.

Make sure there are no bones left in the fish, and no skin. Poach in just enough milk to cover for about 5–10 minutes. Drain the fish, reserving the flavoured milk. Break the fish into pieces.

Peel the potatoes, cut into even pieces, and boil in water until tender. Mash until smooth with the butter or margarine.

Meanwhile, cook the sweetcorn and peas in boiling water for about 5 minutes then drain. Put the fish, sweetcorn, peas and parsley into a deep dish. Grate the cheese for the sauce.

Make the sauce by melting the butter or margarine in a saucepan. Add the flour and stir to combine. When sandy in colour and texture, add the reserved fishy milk and the pint of milk, whisking all the time. When thickened, stir in the mustard and most of the cheese.

Pour the sauce over the fish mixture and top with the mashed potato. Sprinkle with the remaining cheese. Cook in the preheated oven until golden brown, about 20 minutes.

Fish Cakes

These are versatile because you can use a variety of fish. You can also make them the day before, keep them in the fridge (covered), and then fry them when you get home.

Serves 4		Serves 96
450g (1lb)	tuna, cod or haddock fillets	*5.4kg (12lb)*
450g (1lb)	potatoes	*5.4kg (12lb)*
2–3 tablespoons	milk, warmed	*520ml (19fl oz)*
2	eggs	*24*
2 tablespoons	chopped parsley	*10 tablespoons*
	plain flour	
115g (4oz)	fresh breadcrumbs	*1.3kg (3lb)*
	olive oil	
1	lemon (optional)	*12*

Place the fish in a pan and add sufficient water to just cover. Bring to the boil, lower the heat and poach gently for 15 minutes or until just cooked. Cool, then drain the fish and flake, discarding any bones or skin.

Meanwhile, peel the potatoes, cut into even-sized pieces and cook in boiling water until tender. Drain well and mash with enough warm milk to make them smooth. Beat the eggs.

Mix the fish with the mashed potato, parsley, and just enough beaten egg to bind the mixture; it must be firm enough to shape.

With floured hands, shape the mixture into eight (or 96) cakes. Brush with the remaining beaten egg and coat in the breadcrumbs, making sure the cake is covered. Chill for about 30 minutes or until ready to cook.

Heat some oil in a frying pan and shallow-fry the fish cakes, in batches if necessary, for about 5 minutes on each side or until golden and crisp. Drain on kitchen paper then serve immediately, accompanied by lemon wedges if you like.

To bake in the oven, lightly brush with a little olive oil, place on a baking sheet and cook in the oven at 200°C/400°F/Gas 6 for 15–20 minutes or until piping hot and golden brown.

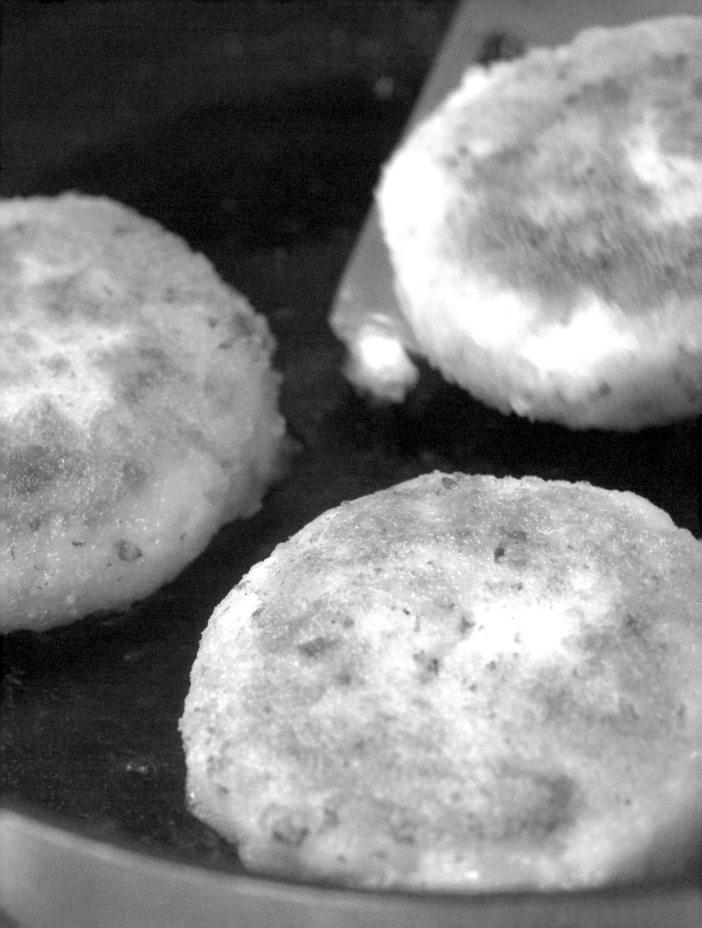

Kedgeree

I love this recipe, but, unfortunately, because of my high numbers, I cannot cook it very often. Try to find undyed smoked haddock. It is a pale, subtle colour, not sunshine dayglo yellow. A green vegetable, such as peas, is a good accompaniment.

Serves 4		Serves 96
450g (1lb)	smoked haddock	5.4kg (12lb)
300ml (10fl oz)	milk	1.2 litres (2 pints)
4	eggs	48
55g (2oz)	onions	675g (1½lb)
1.2 litres (2 pints)	good chicken stock	14 litres (24 pints)
55g (2oz)	butter or margarine	675g (1½lb)
½ teaspoon	mild curry powder	6 teaspoons
450g (1lb)	basmati rice	5.4kg (12lb)

Poach the fish in the milk for about 10 minutes, then drain (discard the milk). Meanwhile, hard-boil the eggs for about 8 minutes then, when cool, shell and roughly chop. Peel and chop the onions. Heat the stock.

In a large saucepan, cook the onion in the butter or margarine until softened, then add the curry powder and rice. Stir to coat the rice in the fat. Add the stock and bring to the boil, then turn down the heat and simmer until the liquid is absorbed, about 10–12 minutes.

When the rice is cooked, stir in the flaked fish with a fork, and add the chopped eggs.

❝I used to bring sandwiches, but now I always have dinners. They're a lot better.❞
SCOTT THURMAN, 9

Tuna Pasta Bake

This is a firm favourite with the children and teaching staff alike. And it's so easy to make, even my youngest son will attempt it. (PS. He's eighteen!)

Serves 4		Serves 96
225g (8oz)	spring onions	900g (2lb)
	olive oil	
2 x 185g cans	tuna in brine	12 x 185g cans
225g (8oz)	frozen peas	2kg (4½lb)
450g (1lb)	dried pasta	5.4kg (12lb)
	Cheese sauce	
115g (4oz)	Cheddar cheese	1.3kg (3lb)
25g (1oz)	butter or margarine	350g (12oz)
25g (1oz)	plain flour	350g (12oz)
600ml (1 pint)	milk	6.8 litres (12 pints)
a pinch	cayenne pepper	½ teaspoon

Preheat the oven to 160°C/325°F/Gas 3.

Cut the green of the spring onions into 5mm (¼in) lengths, and finely slice the remaining white onion. Stir-fry the spring onions for 1–2 minutes in a little oil.

Drain the tuna well, and flake into a bowl. Grate the cheese for the sauce.

Cook the peas in boiling water until tender, about 5 minutes. In a large saucepan of boiling water, cook the pasta until al dente.

To make the sauce, melt the butter or margarine, add the flour and cook until sandy in colour and texture. Add the milk, whisking all the time, and when it is smooth and has thickened, add the cheese, keeping a little back for the topping. Stir in the cayenne.

Mix the pasta, peas, spring onion, tuna and cheese sauce in a deep dish, sprinkle with the remaining grated cheese and bake in the preheated oven until golden on top, about 25 minutes.

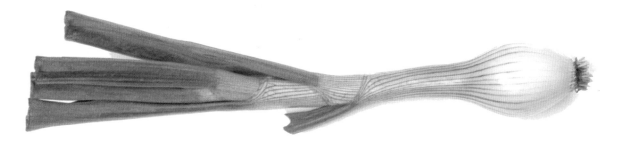

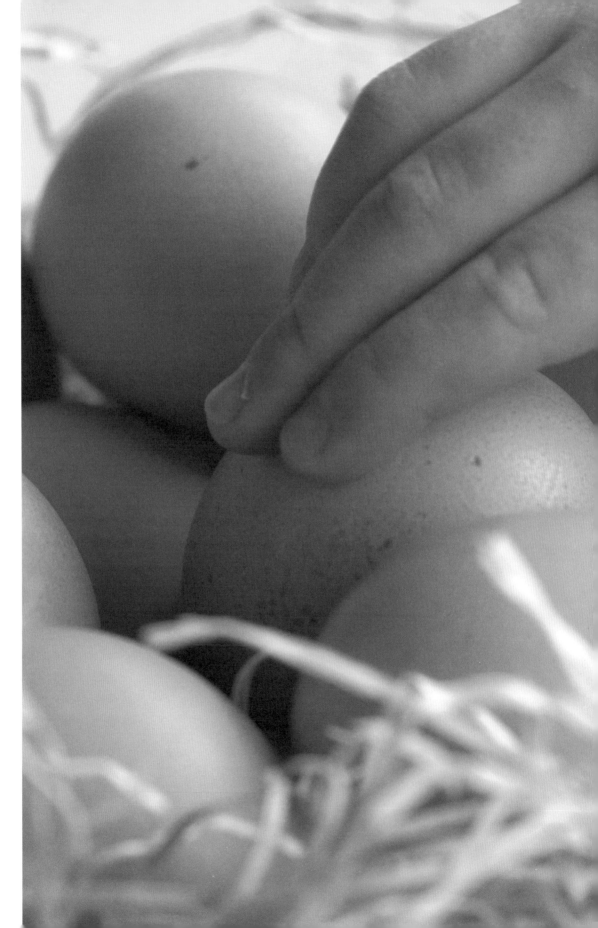

Aussie Pie

I went on holiday to Australia last year, and came across this recipe, which I have adapted slightly. It is a substantial meal in itself, and full of protein, but you could serve it with vegetables as well.

Serves 4		Serves 96
4	eggs	*48*
900g (2lb)	potatoes	*10.8kg (24lb)*
	Cheese sauce	
175g (6oz)	Cheddar cheese	*2kg (4½lb)*
20g (³/₄oz)	butter or margarine	*250g (9oz)*
20g (³/₄oz)	plain flour	*250g (9oz)*
425ml (15fl oz)	milk	*5 litres (9 pints)*

Preheat the oven to 200°C/400°F/Gas 6.

Cook the eggs in boiling water for about 6 minutes, then drain and run under cold running water. Remove the shell and cut into thick slices. Peel and cook the potatoes until soft, then mash until smooth. Grate the cheese for the sauce.

To make the sauce, melt the butter or margarine in a pan, then add the flour and cook until sandy in colour and texture. Add the milk gradually, whisking all the time. Continue to cook until the sauce thickens, then add the cheese.

In a deep tin – about 23cm (9in) square – put a layer of mashed potato then a layer of sliced egg. Continue until you finish with a layer of potato. Pour over the cheese sauce, and bake in the preheated oven until golden brown, about 20 minutes.

❝ There's a fantastic choice and it's healthy food –
the sort of thing that I would feed my kids at home.
As a bonus, the kids seem to love it. **❞**

A MUM

Cheesy Yorkshire Puddings

When I make these, I always leave the batter mixture to rest for about 20 minutes. Then, just before I put the liquid into the tin, I give the batter one last whisk. The puddings always seem to rise better this way – try it! The home-kitchen quantity makes about 24 small puddings. Serve with some good local sausages, mashed potato and seasonal vegetables.

Serves 4		Serves 96
225g (8oz)	plain flour	2.7kg (6lb)
a pinch	ground pepper	½ teaspoon
2	eggs	24
600ml (1 pint)	milk	6.8 litres (12 pints)
115g (4oz)	Cheddar cheese	1.3kg (3lb)
	olive oil	

Sift the flour and pepper together into a bowl. Add the eggs and half the milk, and beat well until smooth. Beat in the remaining milk. Leave to rest for 20 minutes.

Meanwhile, preheat the oven well to 220°C/425°F/Gas 7. Grate the cheese.

Grease patty or Yorkshire pudding tins with olive oil and put into the hot oven for 5 minutes. Take out of the oven and divide the batter mix between the tins. Quickly add a little cheese to each Yorkshire, and bake in the very hot preheated oven until well risen and golden brown, about 10 minutes.

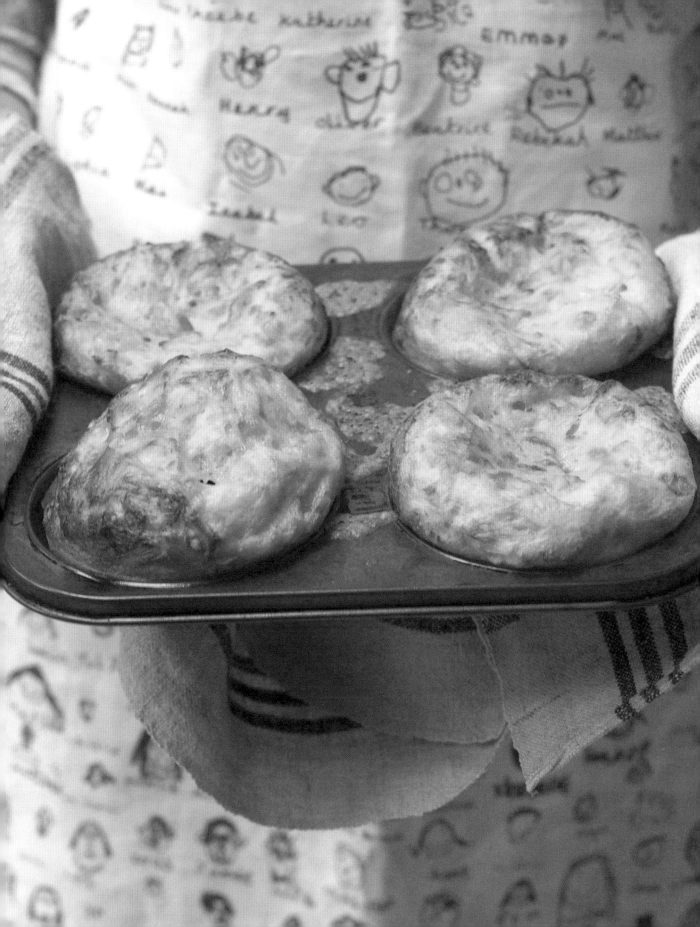

Cheese Puffs

These are quick and easy to make, and another firm favourite with the children. You could also use ready-to-cook or ready-cooked vol-au-vent cases.

Serves 4		*Serves 96*
1 x 500g packet	frozen puff pastry	*12 x 500g packets*
4	eggs	*48*
175g (6oz)	Cheddar cheese	*2kg (4½lb)*
2	tomatoes	*1.3kg (3lb)*
	milk	

Leave the pastry to thaw at room temperature. Preheat the oven to 200°C/400°F/Gas 6.

Hard-boil the eggs for about 6 minutes, then drain and run under cold running water. Remove the shells and cut into thick slices. Grate the cheese, and slice the tomatoes.

Roll the pastry out into a 30cm (12in) square. Cut this square in half. Put most of the cheese along the middle of one piece of the pastry, leaving a little cheese for the top. Put a layer of egg slices then tomato slices on top. Brush the edges of this piece of pastry with water. Fold the remaining piece of pastry in half lengthwise, make a small cut in the middle, and then fold out again on top of the cheese, tomato and egg. Seal the edges well, pressing with your fingers, or with a fork. Brush with milk.

Place on a baking sheet, sprinkle with the remaining cheese, and bake in the preheated oven until golden brown, about 20 minutes. Cut into four large or eight smaller pieces.

❝I like our school dinners because they're healthy for you and warm you up in cold weather. They're much better than they used to be, and I think we're very lucky.❞
LAURA SUTHERLAND, 11

Pasta with Tomato Sauce and Cheese

You could use white or wholemeal pasta for this recipe. The wholemeal will take slightly longer to cook. Dinner ladies don't usually have grills, so they might have to put this in a medium oven to brown.

Serves 4		*Serves 96*
225g (8oz)	Cheddar cheese	*2.25kg (5lb)*
450g (1lb)	shell pasta	*5.4kg (12lb)*
	Tomato sauce	
225g (8oz)	onions	*2kg (4½lb)*
225g (8oz)	carrots	*2kg (4½lb)*
225g (8oz)	celery	*2kg (4½lb)*
225g (8oz)	cherry tomatoes	*2kg (4½lb)*
25g (1oz)	butter or margarine	*350g (12oz)*
115g (4oz)	tomato purée	*1.3kg (3lb)*
850ml (1½ pints)	water	*8.5 litres (15 pints)*

Grate the cheese. Peel and finely chop the onions and carrots. Finely chop the celery, and halve the cherry tomatoes.

Melt the butter or margarine in a saucepan and gently fry the onion, carrot and celery until nearly soft, about 10 minutes. Add the tomato purée and cook for a couple of minutes, then add the cherry tomatoes and water. Stir well, and allow to simmer, covered, until the vegetables are cooked, about a further 20 minutes.

Meanwhile cook the pasta in boiling water until al dente. Drain well. Preheat the grill.

Place the pasta in a casserole dish, cover with the tomato sauce, and sprinkle with the grated cheese. Place under the hot grill until the cheese is golden brown and bubbling, about 10 minutes.

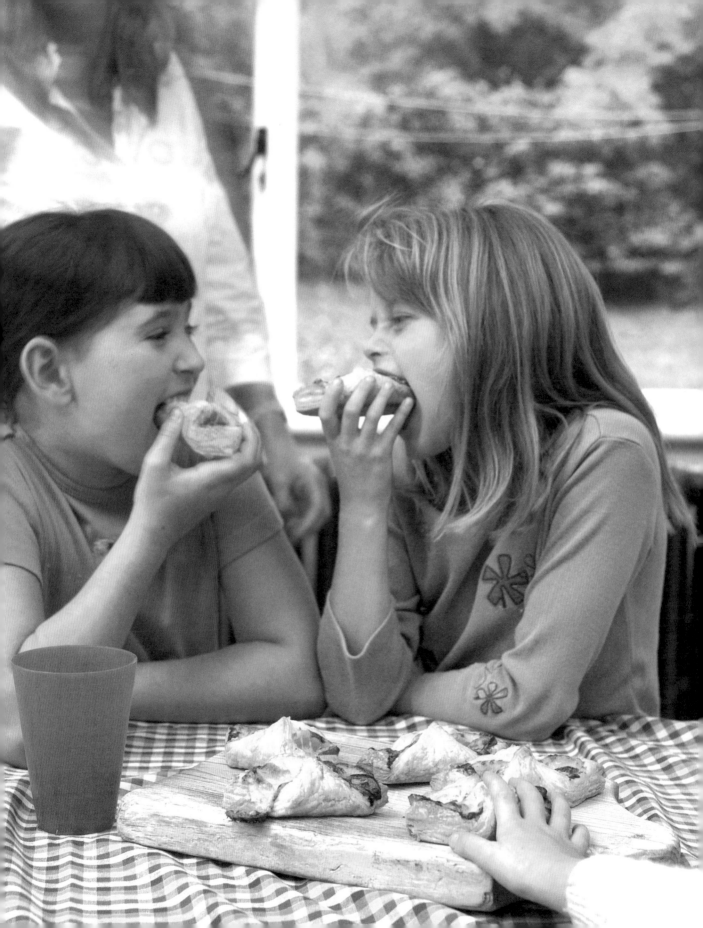

Cheese Triangles with Tomato Sauce

These are easy to make, and the children like them very much, especially when served with this slightly different tomato sauce. You could use ready-to-cook or ready-cooked vol-au-vent cases instead of pastry squares.

Serves 4		Serves 96
1 x 500g packet	frozen puff pastry	12 x 500g packets
225g (8oz)	Cheddar cheese	2.7kg (6lb)
	Tomato sauce	
115g (4oz)	onions	900g (2lb)
1 teaspoon	olive oil	2 tablespoons
25g (1oz)	butter or margarine	350g (12oz)
25g (1oz)	plain flour	350g (12 oz)
115g (4oz)	tomato purée	1.3kg (3lb)
450ml (16fl oz)	water	6.8 litres (12 pints)
1 tablespoon	malt vinegar	175ml (6fl oz)
15g (½oz)	caster sugar	175g (6oz)

Leave the pastry to thaw at room temperature. Preheat the oven to 200°C/400°F/Gas 6.

Make the tomato sauce first. Peel and slice the onions, then fry in the olive oil until softened. Meanwhile, melt the butter or margarine, then add the flour and cook, stirring, until sandy in colour. In a bowl mix the tomato purée with the water, then add to the butter-and-flour roux, stirring all the time until thickened. Then add the vinegar, sugar and onions and cook for a further 5–10 minutes, stirring continuously.

Roll out the defrosted puff pastry and cut it into eight equal-sized squares. Grate the cheese and divide it between the middles of the pastry squares. Fold opposite corners together to make triangles, pressing the sides to seal. Put on a baking sheet and bake in the preheated oven until golden brown, about 10–15 minutes.

With the vol-au-vent cases, if uncooked, bake in the oven for the recommended time (check the packet). Put the cheese in the middle and heat through in the preheated oven until the cheese has melted, about 5 minutes.

Serve the pastries with the warmed tomato sauce.

Macaroni Cheese

Another big hit from our kitchen – the kids seem to love this. Charlie, aged ten, couldn't make up his mind which to have, spaghetti bolognaise or macaroni cheese, when they were both on the menu. I gave him both. I think I may have set a precedent!

Serves 4		Serves 96
225g (8oz)	macaroni	*2.7kg (6lb)*
	olive oil	
Cheese sauce		
225g (8oz)	Cheddar cheese	*2.7kg (6lb)*
85g (3oz)	butter or margarine	*1kg (2¼lb)*
85g (3oz)	plain flour	*1kg (2¼lb)*
1.2 litres (2 pints)	milk	*13.7 litres (24 pints)*
1 teaspoon	wholegrain mustard	*2 tablespoons*

Preheat the oven to 200°C/400°F/Gas 6.

Cook the macaroni in boiling water until just soft, about 9 minutes. Drain, sprinkle with a little olive oil to stop it sticking together, and set to one side.

For the cheese sauce, grate the cheese. Melt the butter or margarine, add the flour, and cook until it changes to a light sandy colour. Add the milk gradually, mixing continuously until smooth, then cook until it starts to thicken. Now, off the heat, add most of the cheese, reserving a quarter for the topping, then the mustard.

Pour the macaroni into a large, ovenproof bowl followed by the cheese sauce, and stir thoroughly. Sprinkle with the remaining cheese. Bake in the preheated oven until golden and bubbling, about 20 minutes.

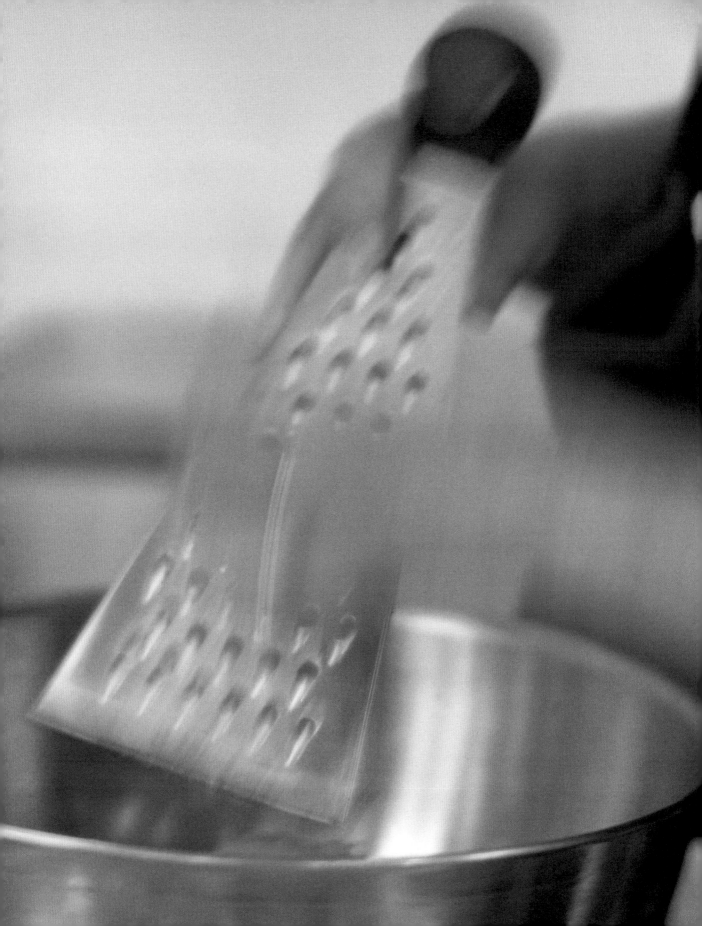

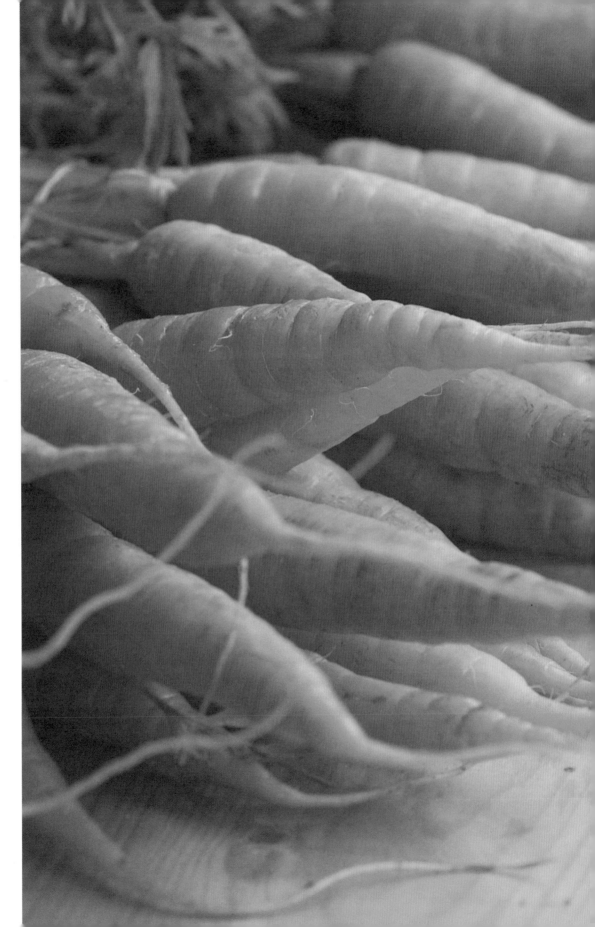

Vegetables and Salads

Vegetable Lasagne

This is a good way to get children to eat vegetables. Make sure you dice them very small and to begin with just give them a small amount. They will be back for more, I can tell you. Serve with some fresh bread rolls or crusty bread.

Serves 4		Serves 96
225g (8oz)	pre-cooked lasagne	2kg (4½lb)
1 tablespoon	olive oil	175ml (6fl oz)
175g (6oz)	onions	1.3kg (3lb)
175g (6oz)	carrots	1.3kg (3lb)
3 sticks	celery	2 heads
175g (6oz)	courgettes	1.3kg (3lb)
½ teaspoon	mixed dried herbs	55g (2oz)
1 x 400g can	chopped tomatoes	2 x A10 (2.7kg) cans
115g (4oz)	tomato purée	1.3kg (3lb)
300ml (10fl oz)	water	3.4 litres (6 pints)
	Cheese sauce	
115g (4oz)	Cheddar cheese	1.3kg (3lb)
25g (1oz)	butter or margarine	350g (12oz)
25g (1oz)	plain flour	350g (12oz)
600ml (1 pint)	milk	6.8 litres (12 pints)
½ teaspoon	wholegrain mustard	55g (2oz)

Preheat the oven to 200°C/400°F/Gas 6. Grease a deep lasagne dish, approximately 30cm (12in) square, with a little of the oil.

Peel and dice the onions. Wash the carrots and celery and then dice. Trim the courgettes, and slice thinly. Grate the cheese for the sauce.

Sauté the onions, carrots, celery and courgettes in the remaining olive oil for a few minutes, then add the herbs, tomatoes, tomato purée and water. Bubble for 10–15 minutes.

Make the cheese sauce by melting the butter or margarine then adding the flour. Cook until the texture and colour are sandy, then add the milk, stirring continuously until thickened and smooth. Add the cheese and mustard, and cook for a further 2–3 minutes.

Arrange half of the lasagne on the base of the dish. Pour half the vegetables over the lasagne, then top with another layer of lasagne. Top with the remaining vegetables, then pour over the cheese sauce. Bake in the preheated oven until golden brown and the lasagne is soft, about 30–35 minutes.

Crunchy Vegetable Crumble

One of the children at school invited his vegetarian grandfather to have a school lunch. Apparently Grandad had been at rather a good restaurant the night before, and this dish was better than what he'd eaten there! Depending on the season, you can use whatever vegetable is available; the more the merrier. You could use carrots, cauliflower, broccoli, parsnips, sweet potato, pumpkin or squash, peppers, courgettes, leeks.

Serves 4		Serves 96
900g (2lb)	seasonal vegetables	*6.75kg (15lb)*
225g (8oz)	onions	*1.1kg (2¹/₂lb)*
1	garlic clove	*6*
1 tablespoon	olive oil	*175ml (6fl oz)*
	White sauce	
25g (1oz)	butter or margarine	*350g (12oz)*
25g (1oz)	plain flour	*350g (12oz)*
600ml (1 pint)	milk	*6.8 litres (12 pints)*
	Topping	
55g (2oz)	Cheddar cheese	*675g (1¹/₂lb)*
55g (2oz)	plain flour	*2.25kg (5lb)*
25g (1oz)	butter or margarine	*1.3kg (3lb)*
25g (1oz)	oats	*675g (1¹/₂lb)*

Preheat the oven to 200°C/400°F/Gas 6. Prepare the seasonal vegetables as appropriate, and cut into largish pieces. Peel and roughly chop the onions, and peel and crush the garlic. Grate the cheese for the topping.

Put the root vegetables, including the onion and garlic, into a roasting tray, and mix with the oil. Roast in the preheated oven for 15 minutes. If using vegetables such as broccoli or cauliflower, blanch in boiling water for a few minutes.

For the topping, put the flour into a large mixing bowl. Cut the butter or margarine into small cubes and rub into the flour. When it looks like breadcrumbs, add the oats and cheese and mix in. Put to one side.

To make the sauce, melt the butter or margarine in a pan, then add the flour and cook over a gentle heat until the mixture turns sandy in colour and texture. Gradually add the milk, beating all the time, and cook until the mixture thickens. Continue to cook for a further 5 minutes over a low heat.

Put the vegetables on the bottom of a large, square, deep dish, then add the sauce. Finally sprinkle the topping over the dish. Cover with foil, and bake in the preheated oven for about 15 minutes. Uncover, and bake for another 15–20 minutes or until the cheese topping is bubbling and golden. Serve with warm crusty bread. Delicious!

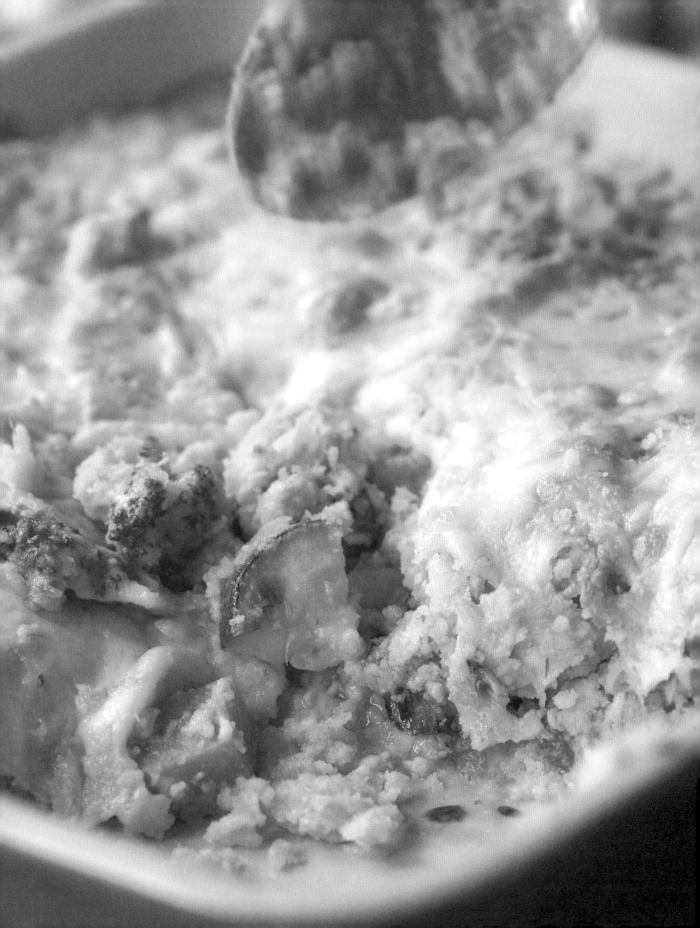

Vegetarian Beanburgers

Dinner ladies, you'll have to make this recipe in batches in the food processor. Serve the burgers in split burger buns, accompanied by tomato relish (see page 208).

Serves 4		Serves 96
2 x 400g cans	red kidney beans	*2 x A10 (2.6kg) cans*
2 x 400g cans	butter beans	*2 x A10 (2.6kg) cans*
1	large onion	*12*
1	garlic clove	*5*
	olive oil	
1 teaspoon	dried thyme	*2 tablespoons*
85g (3oz)	fresh breadcrumbs	*1kg (2¼lb)*
2 tablespoons	soy sauce	*300ml (10fl oz)*
2 tablespoons	lemon juice	*300ml (10fl oz)*

Drain and rinse both types of bean. Peel and finely chop the onion and garlic.

Heat a little oil in a frying pan and fry the onion, garlic and thyme for 10 minutes until softened. Add the beans and fry for a further 5 minutes.

Spoon into a food processor, and pulse briefly to form a rough paste. Transfer the bean mixture to a bowl and stir in the breadcrumbs, soy sauce and lemon juice.

Divide the mixture into eight (or 96) equal portions and shape into burgers. Heat a little oil in a heavy-based frying pan and fry the burgers in batches for 2–3 minutes on each side until golden and cooked through.

Drain the burgers on kitchen paper and keep warm while cooking the remainder.

" I like the meals here because they're tasty, and it isn't sausages and burgers every day, like some children get. "
AMY THORNTON, 11

Cauliflower Cheese

When good local cauliflowers are in season, this is a super dish. It has taken me a long time to get the children to eat this, but now a lot of them love it. You have to persevere …

Serves 4		Serves 96
1 large or 2 small	cauliflower	*12 large or 24 small*
	Cheese sauce	
225g (8oz)	Cheddar cheese	*2.7kg (6lb)*
55g (2oz)	butter or margarine	*675g (1¹/₂lb)*
55g (2oz)	plain flour	*450g (1lb)*
1.2 litres (2 pints)	milk	*12 litres (20 pints)*
¹/₂ teaspoon	wholegrain mustard	*55g (2oz)*

Trim and prepare the cauliflower, and cut into florets – or leave whole (after removing the centre stalk core and cutting a cross in what core is left). Add to boiling water, and cook until nearly ready, but still firm, about 10 minutes. Drain very thoroughly and put into a warmed heatproof dish.

To make the cheese sauce, grate the cheese first. Melt the butter or margarine, then add the flour and cook over a gentle heat until the mixture turns sandy in texture and colour. Gradually add the milk, stirring all the time, and cook until thickened. Off the heat, stir in three-quarters of the cheese and all the mustard.

Pour the cheese sauce over the cauliflower. Sprinkle with the remaining cheese and put under a preheated grill until bubbling and golden, about 4–5 minutes. Dinner ladies would have to put it into a moderate oven to brown.

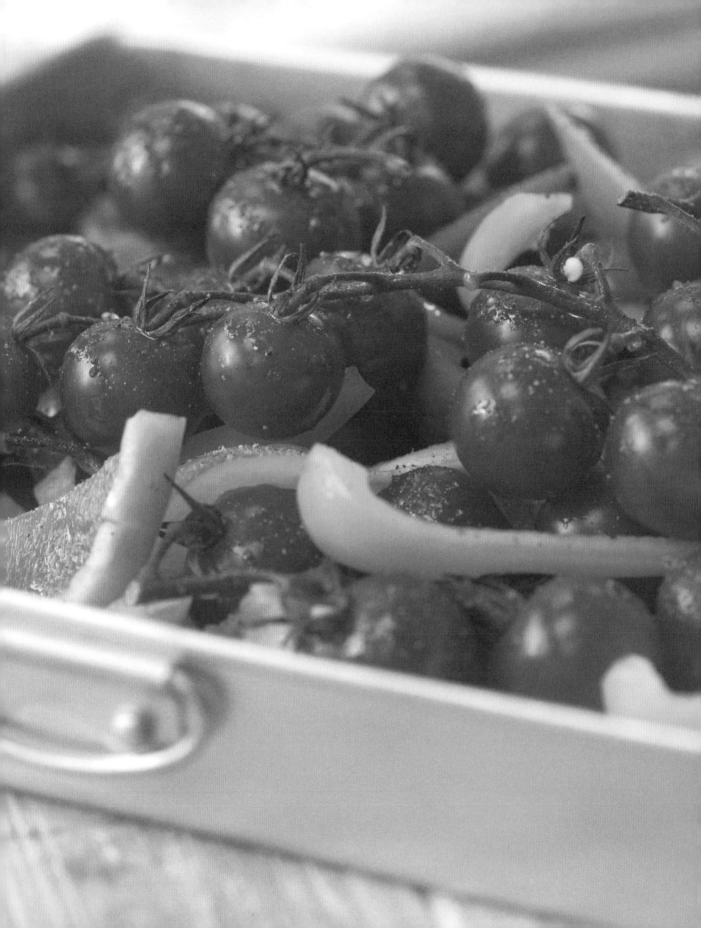

Roasted Cherry Tomatoes

The children seem to love these tomatoes, which they eat as an accompaniment to things like roast lamb or meatballs. I sometimes add peppers as well, as you can see in the photograph, before the dish goes into the oven.

Serves 4		Serves 96
675g (1½lb)	cherry tomatoes	8kg (18lb)
1	green pepper	6
1	yellow pepper	6
1½ tablespoons	olive oil	200ml (7fl oz)

Preheat the oven to 200°C/400°F/Gas 6.

Wash the tomatoes. Halve the peppers, seed them, and cut the flesh into strips.

Pour the olive oil into a large deep tin, and put into the preheated oven to warm through. Add the tomatoes and pepper strips and roast until soft and brown, about 10 minutes.

**"The dinner was brilliant.
My Dad does most of the cooking at home but
we all thought today's school dinner was much better
than anything he can come up with. "**
NAOMI MOSS, 11

Tagliatelle with Summer Vegetables

This vegetarian dish uses the tomato sauce from the chicken meatballs recipe on page 124. The tomato sauce could simply be added to pasta and served with grated Parmesan or Cheddar, but it's nice to make it more substantial using fresh vegetables. Choose summer vegetables such as courgettes, French beans, peas, cherry tomatoes and broad beans.

Serves 4		Serves 96
700g (1lb 9oz)	summer vegetables	8.4kg (18½lb)
1	onion	6
1	garlic clove	6
1 tablespoon	olive oil	175ml (6fl oz)
	fresh tomato sauce (see page 124)	
450g (1lb)	tagliatelle	5.4kg (12lb)
	Cheddar cheese (optional)	

Prepare the vegetables as appropriate. Blanch vegetables such as courgettes, French beans, broad beans and peas in boiling water for 1–2 minutes, drain and immediately refresh in cold water.

Peel and finely chop the onion, and peel and crush the garlic. Heat the oil in a large frying pan and cook the onion and garlic for 2–3 minutes. Add the blanched vegetables and others like halved cherry tomatoes, and cook over a gentle heat for 1 minute. Add the tomato sauce and stir until bubbling.

Cook the tagliatelle in a large pan of boiling water until al dente, about 10–11 minutes. Drain, reserving 4 tablespoons of the cooking water. Return the pasta and reserved water to the large pan and add the vegetables in tomato sauce. Serve at once, with grated cheese if you like.

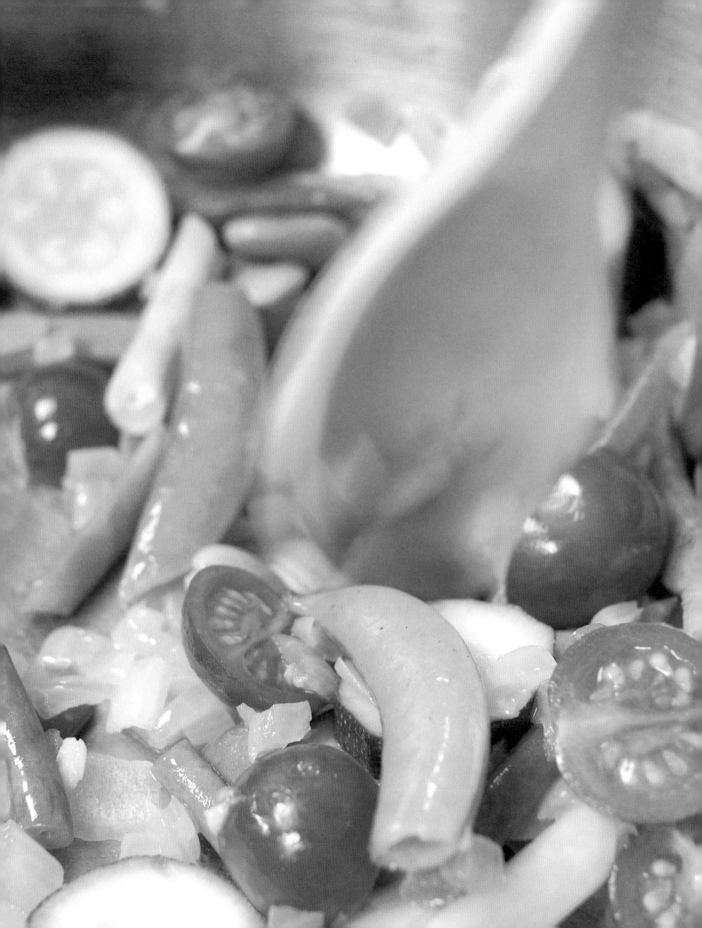

Sneaky Pie

I have called this pie 'sneaky' because of the veg it has in it. They are 'hidden' in the baked beans. Use low sugar and salt baked beans.

Serves 4		Serves 96
	Pastry	
225g (8oz)	plain flour	2.7kg (6lb)
a pinch	cayenne pepper	2 teaspoons
55g (2oz)	margarine	675g (1½lb)
55g (2oz)	vegetable shortening	675g (1½lb)
25ml (1fl oz)	water	350ml (12fl oz)
	Filling and topping	
900g (2lb)	potatoes	10.8kg (24lb)
50ml (2fl oz)	warm milk	300ml (10fl oz)
25g (1oz)	butter or margarine	300g (10½oz)
1 small	onion	675g (1½lb)
1	carrot	1.3kg (3lb)
1	courgette	12
½	red pepper	6
½	green pepper	6
	olive oil	
1 x 400g can	baked beans	1 x A10 (2.6kg) can
115g (4oz)	Cheddar cheese (optional)	1.3kg (3lb)

Preheat the oven to 160°C/325°F/Gas 3.

For the pastry, sift the flour and cayenne pepper into a bowl. Cut the margarine and vegetable shortening into cubes, add to the flour, and rub in until the mixture resembles breadcrumbs. Add the water and mix with a knife until you have a dough. Wrap in clingfilm and put in the fridge to chill, before rolling it out and using it to line a 20–23cm (8–9in) flan tin. Neaten the edges and bake blind (lined with foil and baking beans or dried beans) in the preheated oven for about 15–20 minutes. Remove, and turn the oven up to 200°C/400°F/Gas 6.

Peel the potatoes and cook in boiling water for about 15–20 minutes. Drain and mash the potatoes with the warm milk until very smooth, then add the butter or margarine.

Peel the onion and carrot. Trim the courgette, and seed the peppers. Dice all the vegetables into small pieces, and sweat to soften in a little olive oil.

Pour the baked beans into the flan case then layer the vegetables over them. Finally smooth the potato on the top. You can sprinkle a little grated cheese over the flan if liked. Bake in the hot oven for about 20 minutes.

Rainbow salad

We serve this colourful salad in summer.

Serves 4		Serves 96
225g (8oz)	long-grain rice	1.3kg (3lb)
1	red pepper	900g (2lb)
1 small	onion	900g (2lb)
55g (2oz)	frozen peas	450g (1lb)
55g (2oz)	frozen sweetcorn	450g (1lb)
1 tablespoon	olive oil	175ml (6fl oz)

Place the rice in a sieve and rinse under cold running water. Bring a pan of water to the boil, add the rice, and return to the boil. Stir once then reduce the heat, cover and simmer for about 11 minutes or until tender. Drain in a sieve and rinse with cold water, then allow to cool.

Seed and finely chop the pepper. Peel the onion and finely chop. Bring a small pan of water to the boil and add the pepper, onion, peas and sweetcorn. Bring back to the boil and cook for 2 minutes. Drain and set aside to cool.

Combine all the ingredients in a large bowl and drizzle with the olive oil.

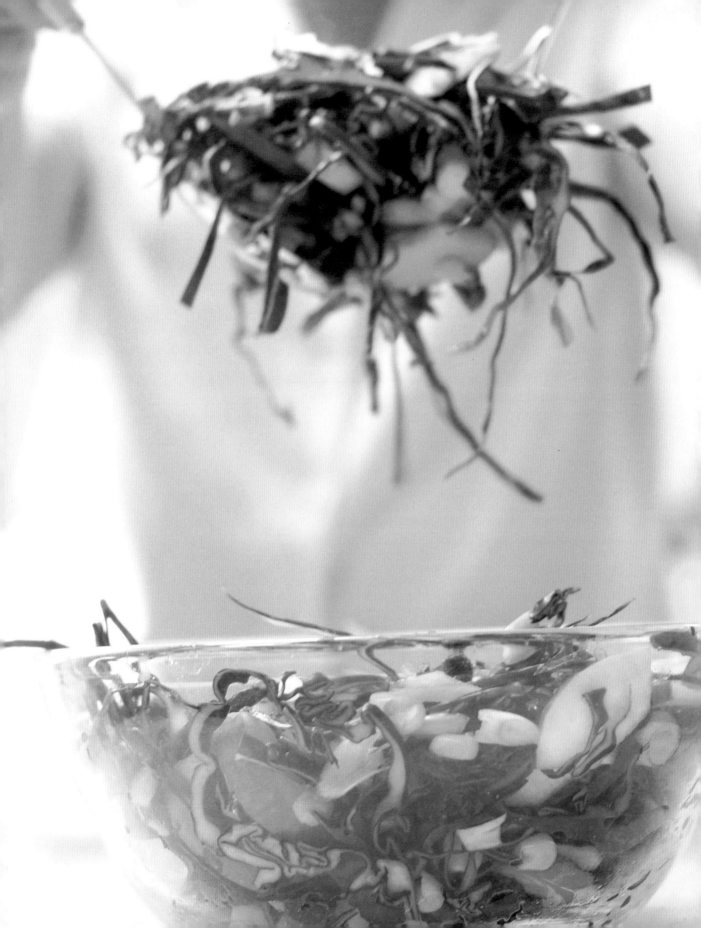

St Peter's Salad

At St Peter's throughout the year we always have a salad table, where the children can help themselves to as little or as much as they like. This salad is good in the autumn, when local eating apples are at their best. It can be made up to 5 hours in advance; cover and chill.

Serves 4		Serves 96
175g (6oz)	frozen sweetcorn	1.8kg (4lb)
250g (9oz)	red cabbage	2.7kg (6lb)
1 bunch	spring onions	5 bunches
225g (8oz)	eating apples	2.7kg (6lb)
115g (4oz)	sultanas	450g (1lb)
25ml (1fl oz)	mayonnaise	350ml (12fl oz)

Bring a small saucepan of water to the boil, add the sweetcorn, and bring back to the boil. Simmer for 2 minutes, drain and leave to go cold.

Wash and shred the cabbage finely, and put into a large mixing bowl. Trim the onions, discarding outside leaves, then slice them finely. Wash and core the apples, and dice them. Add the onion and apple to the cabbage in the bowl, with the cold sweetcorn and sultanas.

Mix all the ingredients together with the mayonnaise.

❝They're really good because we wouldn't normally get all this and they're really cheap.❞

LAURA CREE, 9

Pasta and Sweetcorn Salad

There is something about pasta and sweetcorn together that children love. Perhaps it has to do with the idea that you eat first with your eyes! You can make this a day ahead; cover and chill.

Serves 4		Serves 96
225g (8oz)	tricoloured pasta	*2.7kg (6lb)*
175g (6oz)	frozen sweetcorn	*2kg (4½lb)*
1 tablespoon	olive oil	*175ml (6fl oz)*

Bring a large pan of water to the boil, add the pasta and bring back to the boil. Reduce the heat and cook for about 10 minutes or until the pasta is al dente. Drain through a sieve, rinse with boiling water and allow to cool.

Bring a small pan of water to the boil and cook the sweetcorn for 2–3 minutes, then drain.

When the sweetcorn and pasta are cool, mix together in a large bowl and drizzle with the olive oil.

❝ The dinners are brilliant. They're a little bit different to how they used to be when I started. ❞
MYLES EVANS, 11

California Salad

I like to make my own mayonnaise, but there are some good ready-made versions available. This salad is colourful, with good texture and flavour. It also has an interesting name – which, for some children, might suggest Hollywood and Disneyland! You can prepare the tomato, cucumber and celery up to a day in advance; add the bananas, apple and mayonnaise just before serving.

Serves 4		Serves 96
115g (4oz)	tomatoes	1.3kg (3lb)
½	cucumber	6
4 sticks	celery	2 heads
2	bananas	2.25kg (5lb)
1	red apple	1.3kg (3lb)
½	lemon	6
1 tablespoon	mayonnaise	300ml (10fl oz)

Quarter the tomatoes and remove the seeds, then roughly chop. Cut the cucumber in half lengthways and remove the seeds with a teaspoon. Roughly chop. Cut the celery into thin strips then cut across into fine dice. Set aside in a large bowl.

Peel the bananas and roughly chop. Quarter, core and roughly chop the apple. Put the apple and banana into a small bowl and toss in the lemon juice.

Add the bananas and apple to the remaining ingredients and toss together with the mayonnaise.

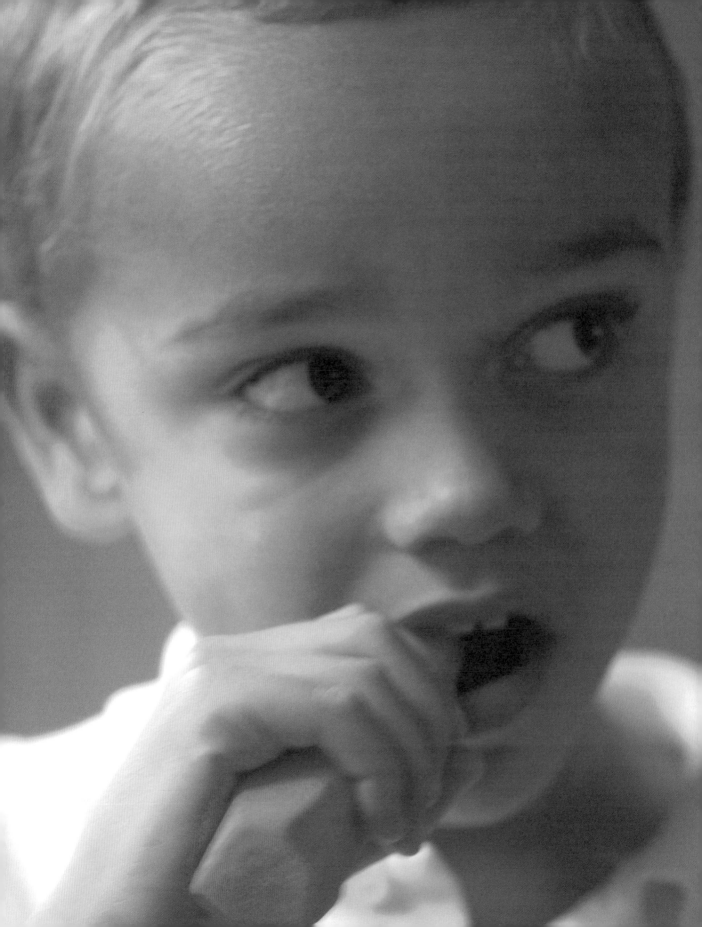

Green Bean, Carrot and Rice Salad

When you are thinking what to do with all those green beans in the garden, get the children to go and pick you some and make this dish.

Serves 4		Serves 96
140g (5oz)	long-grain rice	1.6kg (3½lb)
175g (6oz)	carrots	2kg (4½lb)
140g (5oz)	green beans	1.6kg (3½lb)
1 tablespoon	olive oil	175ml (6fl oz)

Place the rice in a sieve and rinse under cold running water. Bring a large pan of water to the boil, add the rice and bring back to the boil. Stir once then reduce the heat, cover and simmer for about 11 minutes or until the rice is tender. Drain in a sieve and rinse under cold water. Leave to stand until cool.

Meanwhile, peel the carrots and cut into long strips, then cut across to make small dice. Top and tail the green beans then cut each bean into three.

Bring a small pan of water to the boil and cook the carrots and beans for 2 minutes, drain through a sieve then run under cold water to retain the colour of the green beans.

Toss the rice and vegetables with the olive oil and serve.

Bugsy's Salad

The children named this recipe 'Bugsy' because of the carrots. It can be made 3/4 hours ahead of serving, cover and chill.

Serves 4		Serves 96
225g (8oz)	carrots	2.7kg (6lb)
1	orange	12
55g (2oz)	sultanas	450g (1lb)
2 teaspoons	olive oil	6 tablespoons
1 teaspoon	wine vinegar	3 tablespoons

Peel the carrots and grate them thickly into a large bowl. Wash the orange, and grate the zest finely. Remove and discard the pith and chop the orange flesh into chunks. Mix the carrot, orange zest and flesh and sultanas together in a bowl.

Whisk the oil and vinegar to make a dressing. Pour over the carrots, and turn lightly until well mixed together.

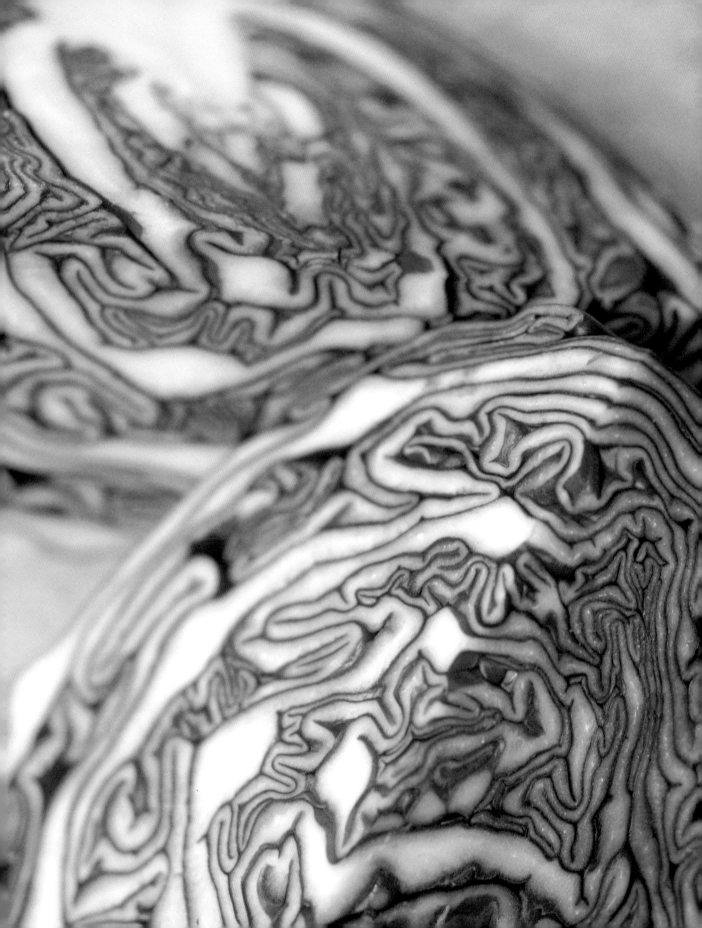

Jane's Coleslaw

Jane makes this every day for the children, and they love it. It can also be made up to a day in advance and kept in the fridge.

Serves 4		Serves 96
250g (9oz)	red cabbage	2.7kg (6lb)
175g (6oz)	carrots	1.8kg (4lb)
2	tomatoes	1.3kg (3lb)
½	cucumber	6
110g (4oz)	dried apricots	900g (2lb)
1 tablespoon	mayonnaise	300ml (10fl oz)

Finely shred the red cabbage and put into a large bowl. Peel and grate the carrots, and add to the bowl.

Quarter the tomatoes and remove the seeds, then chop the flesh roughly. Split the cucumber lengthways and remove the seeds with a teaspoon. Cut into long strips then cut across to make fine dice. Chop the apricots into dice.

Add the tomato, cucumber and apricot to the cabbage and carrot with the mayonnaise, and mix well.

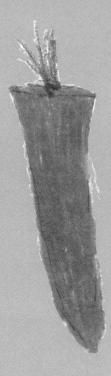

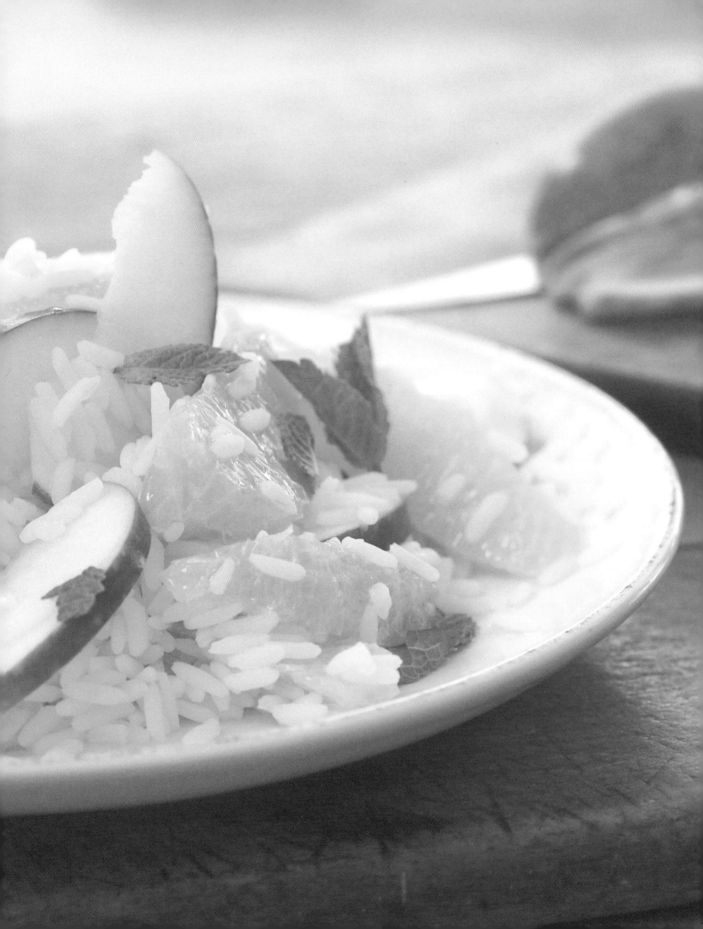

Apple and Orange Salad

This is one way of including fruit in your children's diet.

Serves 4		Serves 96
225g (8oz)	long-grain rice	2.25kg (5lb)
1	eating apple	12
1	orange	12
1 tablespoon	olive oil	175ml (6fl oz)

Place the rice in a sieve and rinse under cold running water. Bring a pan of water to the boil, and add the rice. Bring back to the boil, then cook until tender, about 11 minutes. Rinse in cold water, drain well, and allow to cool.

Wash the apple, quarter and core, then dice or slice. Use a sharp knife to cut away the peel and pith of the orange, then roughly chop the flesh.

Put the rice in a large mixing bowl and stir in the apple and orange, drizzle with olive oil and serve.

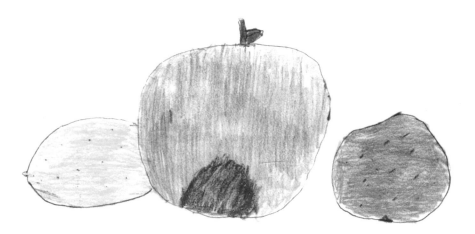

Tomato Relish

This could be a twist on tomato ketchup. It's good served with the vegetarian beanburgers on page 190, or the real chicken nuggets on page 131.

Serves 4		Serves 96
1	large onion	*12*
1	garlic clove	*5*
2 tablespoons	olive oil	*350ml (12fl oz)*
300ml (10fl oz)	tomato passata	*3.4 litres (6 pints)*
1 tablespoon	muscovado sugar	*12 tablespoons*
1 tablespoon	malt vinegar	*12 tablespoons*
2	oranges	*24*
3 medium	ripe tomatoes	*2.7kg (6lb)*

Peel and finely chop the onion, and peel and crush the garlic. Heat the oil in a pan, add the onion and garlic and cook over a low heat for about 10 minutes until the onion has softened. Add the tomato passata with the sugar and vinegar and bring to the boil. Reduce the heat and simmer for 5 minutes.

Meanwhile, peel and segment the oranges, then roughly chop the flesh. Roughly chop the tomatoes. Add the oranges and tomatoes to the sauce and cook for a further 2–3 minutes. Take off the heat, and allow to cool.

" The food here is sometimes organic, which means it's healthier for you. "

HENRY ELLIS, 8

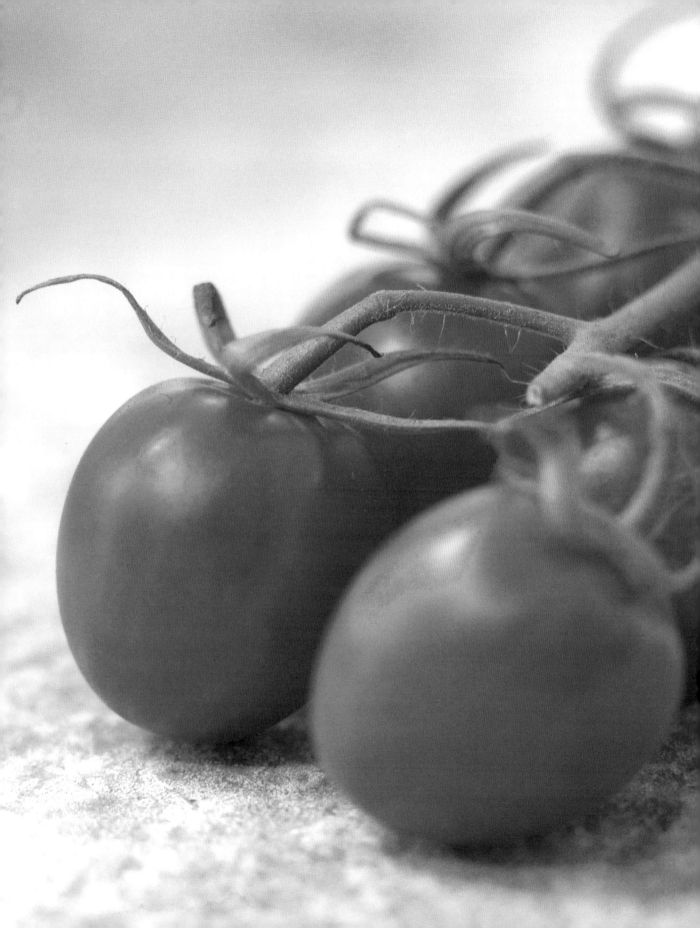

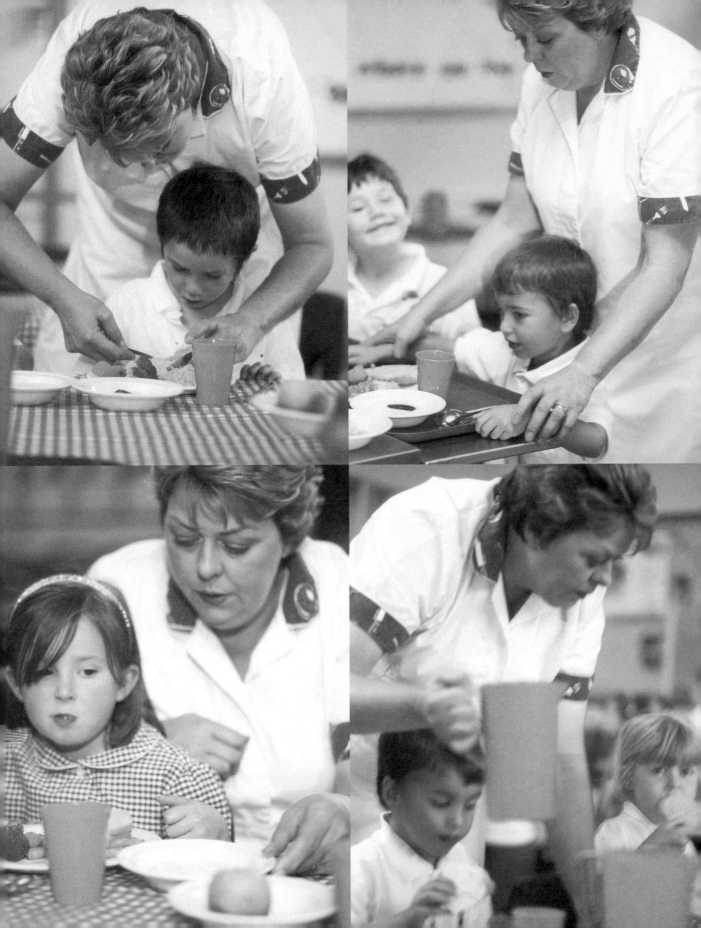

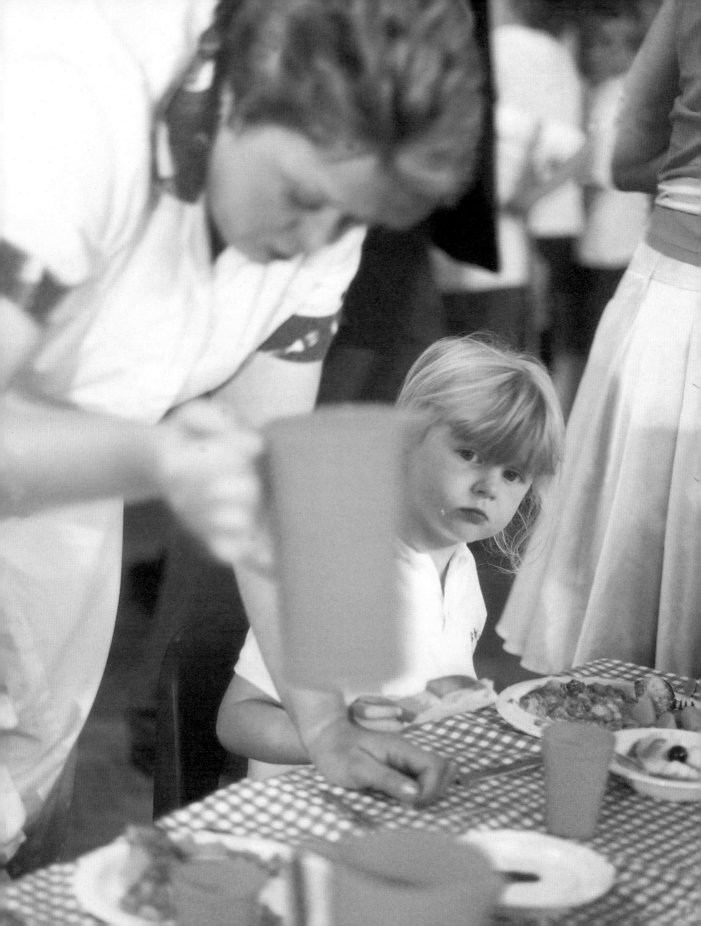

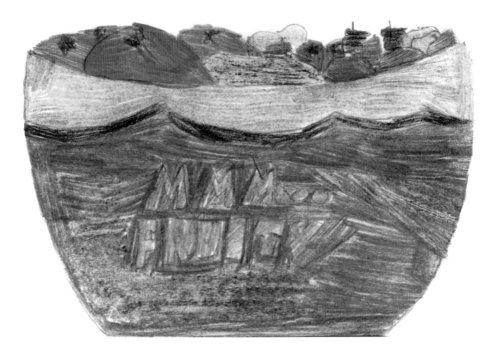

SWEET THINGS ARE NOT vital in the diet – but most of us, particularly children, appreciate sweet flavours. This liking is innate, thought to be a relic of our long-ago ancestors' fruit-eating days – and breast milk, of course, probably the first flavour most of us encounter, is quite sweet.

It's difficult to hit the right balance when serving desserts or puddings, whether at home or school. Many of us think that a savoury course is automatically followed by a sweet one, and children can be prone to eat less of the more valuable protein foods in anticipation of the sweet thing, which they might like better, to come. Very small children, whose calorie requirements are low, could be filled up with sweet things and miss out completely on more nourishing foods. One answer is to serve a sweet course only occasionally, making it a rarity rather than a constant. Two courses are not always necessary.

Always try to make sure that sweet things are made with good ingredients, with organic flours, with eggs, milk, yoghurt and, especially, fruit. Avoid packet puddings, which are always high in sugar (and occasionally, surprisingly, salt). Fruits can be served raw in the hand, and if you choose seasonally, children should never be bored. Fruits taste best in season, too. Or fruits can be cooked, in crumbles, baked, and mixed in with yoghurt. There are quite a few ideas in the following pages, in all of which I have cut down on the original sugar quantities (and I haven't had any complaints).

There are more than a few apple ideas here, but I truly believe that an apple a day keeps the doctor away. For instance, a medium-sized Bramley apple, baked, provides almost half the recommended daily intake of Vitamin C. The pectin in apples – which is what makes them so useful in jam- and jelly-making – is capable of reducing high cholesterol levels. And an apple a day, both for adults and children, exercises the jaws and hardens the gums.

And we can't forget chocolate. I know it can be bad for teeth, and that it contains fat, but it is delicious. I serve something chocolatey every now and again, primarily because the children love it!

And if sweet puddings and desserts can hardly be considered vital in the diet, then cakes, biscuits and scones are certainly not needed. But again, because they are sweet in flavour, they are really appreciated by children – and, in my experience, by half of the staff at St Peter's. Sometimes, especially in summer, we offer baked goods instead of hot puddings. The children like to eat things in their hands, and on the days when they don't have an apple, they might have a biscuit, muffin, scone or slice of cake. They love my chocolate chip cookie days, and I'm always getting asked when I am next going to make my carrot cake.

Making cakes, biscuits and scones is time-consuming, I know, but it's not something you are going to do all that often, and it's fun for the children if they are allowed to become involved. There's a lot even the smallest child can do to help when baking, not least licking out the bowl (one of my prime childhood memories!). And, although the recipes in this chapter may contain sugar, at least you know how much sugar is involved – not something you can be certain of with baked goods. And you can also include a certain amount of fruit when baking – see the recipes for carrot cake, date slice and banana bread, for instance.

Many of the recipes in the following pages can be made for tea – because children can be very hungry when they get home from school. They may have eaten a good lunch – they certainly do when I've got anything to do with it – but after an afternoon of concentration and play, they need something to tide them over until the evening meal.

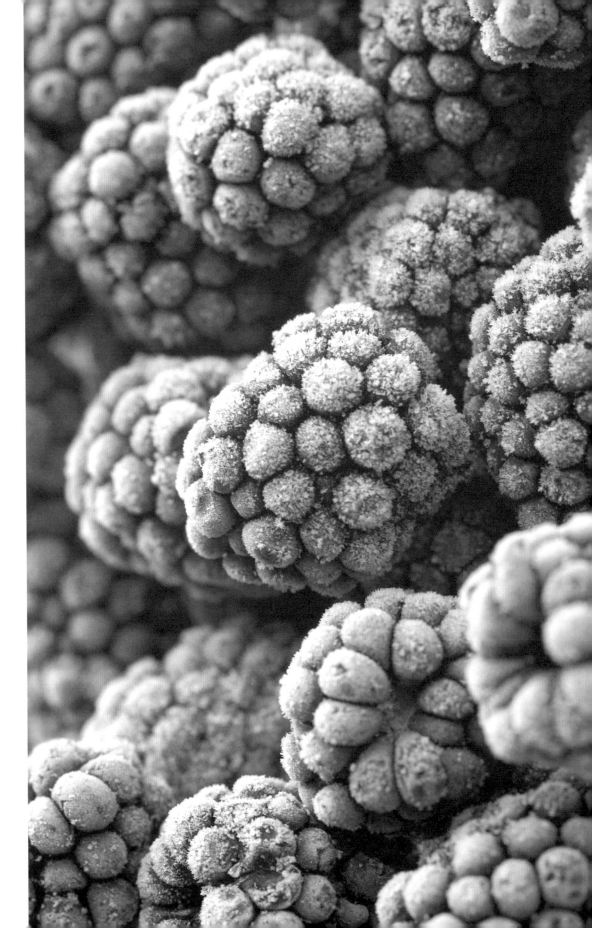

Puddings and Tarts

Apple and Orange Duff

'Oranges and lemons, say the bells of St Clement's' – but here we are using oranges and apples instead.

Serves 4		Serves 96
225g (8 oz)	plain flour	2.7kg (6lb)
15g (½oz)	baking powder	175g (6oz)
55g (2oz)	butter or margarine	675g (1½lb)
85g (3oz)	caster sugar	900g (2lb)
450g (1lb)	Bramley apples	9kg (20lb)
225g (8oz)	oranges	2.7kg (6lb)
125ml (4fl oz)	milk	1.35 litres (48fl oz)
425ml (15fl oz)	boiling water	5 litres (9 pints)
2 tablespoons	granulated sugar	350g (12oz)

Preheat the oven to 190°C/375°F/Gas 5.

Sift the flour and baking powder into a bowl. Cut the fat into cubes and rub into the flour until the texture is like breadcrumbs. Add 25g (1oz) of the sugar. Kids can help with this bit. (Make sure they wash their hands first!)

Peel, core and slice the apples, and arrange in a deep tin, about 20 cm (8in) square. Sprinkle with the remaining caster sugar. Peel the oranges, carefully removing all the pith, and divide into segments. Arrange in the dish with the apples.

Add enough milk to the flour and butter mixture to give a soft dough that can be flattened by hand. Form into a piece that will cover the tin. Shape the dough so that it fits the tin, just covering the fruit.

Pour the boiling water over the dough in the tin, and dredge with the granulated sugar. Immediately place in the hot oven, and bake until the scone topping is well risen and golden brown, about 35–40 minutes.

Dinner ladies, use 12 tins for the 96 portions, and divide the dough into 12. Only pour water on those tins about to go into the oven at any one time.

Cornflake Tart

This must be remembered by nearly the whole population. Wherever I go, people ask if it is still made, and if it is, could I send them one!

Serves 4		Serves 96
Pastry		
225g (8oz)	plain flour	2.7kg (6lb)
55g (2oz)	margarine	675g (1½lb)
55g (2oz)	vegetable shortening	675g (1½lb)
15g (½oz)	caster sugar	175g (6oz)
25ml (1fl oz)	water	350ml (12fl oz)
Filling		
175g (6oz)	seedless raspberry jam	1.8kg (4lb)
55g (2oz)	butter or margarine	675g (1½lb)
55g (2oz)	caster sugar	675g (1½lb)
25g (1oz)	golden syrup	350g (12oz)
175g (6oz)	cornflakes	1.8kg (4lb)

To make the pastry, sift the flour into a large bowl. Cut the margarine and vegetable shortening into cubes and quickly rub into the flour using your fingertips until the mixture resembles breadcrumbs. Sprinkle in the sugar and water and mix, using a round-bladed knife, until the mixture begins to stick together in large lumps. With one hand, collect the dough together to form a ball. Turn out on to a clean work surface and gently knead and shape into an even ball, then roll out and use to line a 20–23cm (8–9in) loose-based flan tin. Chill for about 30 minutes. Preheat the oven to 200°C/400°F/Gas 6.

Neaten the edges of the pastry, line the pastry case with greaseproof paper, and fill with baking beans (or dried beans). Bake blind in the preheated oven for about 15 minutes. Remove the beans and paper, and return to the oven to dry out for a further 5–10 minutes.

Spread the base of the pastry case with jam.

Melt the butter or margarine, sugar and syrup together in a pan, then add the cornflakes and mix. Spread this on top of the jam in the pastry case, and leave to cool and set.

Rhubarb Crunch

A winter warmer, and an introduction for children to the distinct flavour of rhubarb. The orange and cinnamon help to take the sharpness away. You can use fresh or frozen rhubarb.

Serves 4		Serves 96
450g (1lb)	rhubarb	*9kg (20lb)*
1 piece	orange rind	*10 pieces*
50ml (2fl oz)	water	*900ml (2 pints)*
1 teaspoon	ground cinnamon	*55g (2oz)*
2	eggs	*24*
55g (2oz)	cornflour	*675g (1½lb)*
55g (2oz)	golden syrup	*675g (1½lb)*
475ml (17fl oz)	milk	*5.8 litres (10¼ pints)*

Crumble topping

55g (2oz)	butter or margarine	*675g (1½lb)*
115g (4oz)	rolled oats	*1.3kg (3lb)*
85g (3oz)	brown sugar	*1kg (2¼lb)*

Preheat the oven to 190°C/375°F/Gas 5.

Cut the rhubarb into small pieces, place in a saucepan with the orange rind, cover with the water and simmer until soft, about 5–10 minutes. Remove the orange rind. Place the fruit and its juices in a deep tin and sprinkle with the cinnamon.

Beat the eggs, cornflour and syrup together in a heavy-based pan, and stir in the milk. Place the pan over a low heat and cook, whisking continuously, until the custard has thickened. Cool slightly, then pour over the fruit.

For the crumble, melt the butter or margarine in a pan, stir in the oats and sugar then sprinkle it over the custard. Bake in the preheated oven for about 25 minutes until the crumble mixture is golden.

Apple Pie

I use ovenproof plates to make these, as they look better than tins. It takes longer when I am making enough for the children, but it is worth it. For a change, you could add some sultanas to the apple.

Serves 4		Serves 96
900g (2lb)	Bramley apples	9kg (20lb)
115g (4oz)	caster sugar	900g (2lb)
1 teaspoon	ground cinnamon	55g (2oz)
	Pastry	
450g (1lb)	plain flour	4kg (9lb)
115g (4oz)	margarine	1kg (2¼lb)
115g (4oz)	vegetable shortening	1kg (2¼lb)
15g (½oz)	caster sugar	175g (6oz)
50ml (2fl oz)	water	500ml (18fl oz)

Peel, core and slice the apples. Put in a pan, add a little water and simmer until soft. Remove from the heat and sprinkle with the sugar and cinnamon. Leave to cool.

Make the pastry as described on page 216. Wrap in clingfilm and chill for about 30 minutes. Meanwhile, preheat the oven to 190°C/375°F/Gas 5.

Divide the pastry into two, and roll out one half into a circle slightly larger than a 25cm (10in) heatproof plate. Place on the plate, and put the apple on top. Roll out the remaining pastry to a circle to cover the top of the pie, place on top of the apple, brush the edges with water, and press to seal. Trim, and use any trimmings to make leaves for the top of the pie. Cut a steam vent in the middle, then brush the pastry with water and sprinkle with extra sugar.

Bake in the preheated oven for 35–40 minutes.

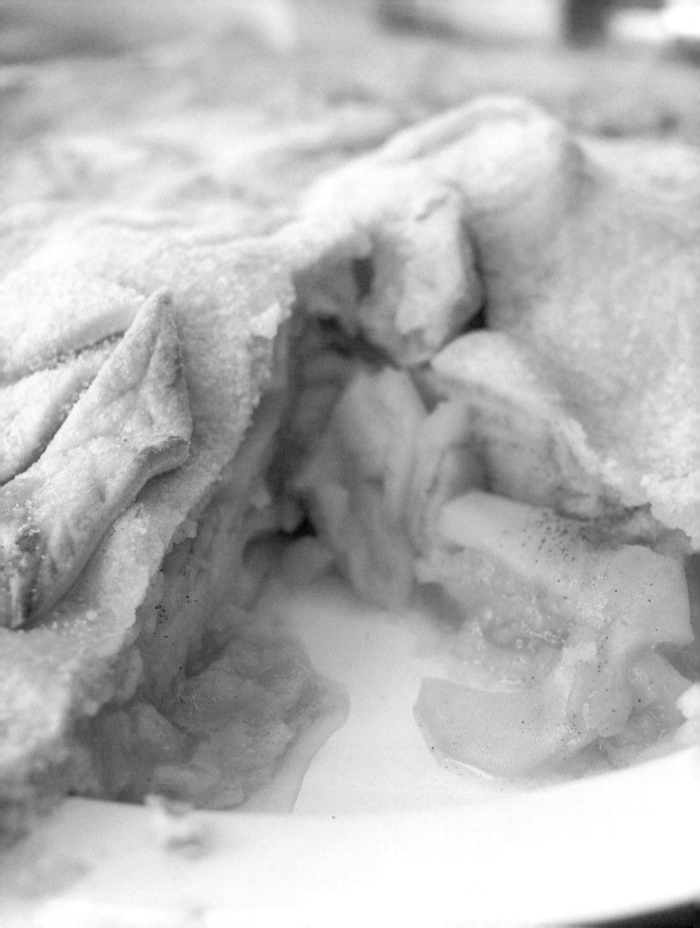

Viennese Tart

This is a larger version of those little Viennese pastries that you can buy.

Serves 4		Serves 96
	Pastry	
225g (8oz)	plain flour	2.7kg (6lb)
55g (2oz)	margarine	675g (1½lb)
55g (2oz)	vegetable shortening	675g (1½lb)
15g (½oz)	caster sugar	175g (6oz)
25ml (1fl oz)	water	350ml (12fl oz)
	Filling	
225g (8oz)	seedless raspberry jam	2.7kg (6lb)
150g (5½oz)	butter or margarine	1.8kg (4lb)
50g (1¾oz)	icing sugar	520g (1lb 3oz)
140g (5oz)	plain flour	1.6kg (3¾lb)
	milk (optional)	

Make the pastry as described on page 216, then roll out and use to line a 20–23cm (8–9in) loose-based flan tin. Chill for about 30 minutes. Preheat the oven to 200°C/400°F/Gas 6.

Trim the pastry edges, then line the pastry case with greaseproof paper, fill with baking beans (or dried beans) and bake blind for 15 minutes. Remove the beans and paper and return to the oven to dry out for a further 5–10 minutes. Remove from the oven, and spread the jam across the base. Reduce the temperature of the oven to 190°C/375°F/Gas 5.

Cream the butter or margarine in a bowl, using a wooden spoon, then add the icing sugar and flour and beat well. You may need to add a little milk as the filling can be quite stiff. Put this in a piping bag fitted with a star tube, and pipe across the jam in a decorative pattern, letting the jam show through.

Bake in the preheated oven for 20 minutes until the pastry is cooked but the topping has not browned.

Gainsborough Tart

I often wonder if this recipe originated in Gainsborough in Lincolnshire, or whether it came from Suffolk, where the famous painter was born and brought up. Perhaps you could let me know.

Serves 4		Serves 96
	Pastry	
225g (8oz)	plain flour	*2.7kg (6lb)*
55g (2oz)	margarine	*675g (1¹/₂lb)*
55g (2oz)	vegetable shortening	*675g (1¹/₂lb)*
15g (¹/₂oz)	caster sugar	*175g (6oz)*
25ml (1fl oz)	water	*350ml (12fl oz)*
	Filling	
175g (6oz)	strawberry jam	*1.8kg (4lb)*
85g (3oz)	butter or margarine	*925g (2lb 1oz)*
85g (3oz)	caster sugar	*925g (2lb 1oz)*
1	egg	*12*
85g (3oz)	ground rice	*925g (2lb 1oz)*
1¹/₂ level teaspoons	baking powder	*40g (1¹/₂oz)*
2 tablespoons	milk	*350ml (12fl oz)*
85g (3oz)	desiccated coconut	*925g (2lb 1oz)*

Make the pastry as described on page 216, then roll out and use to line a 20–23cm (8–9in) loose-based flan tin. Chill for about 30 minutes. Preheat the oven to 200°C/400°F/Gas 6, and put a baking sheet in it to heat up.

Spread the base of the pastry case with jam.

Cream the butter or margarine and sugar together, then add the beaten egg. Mix the ground rice and baking powder together, and stir into the creamed mixture. Mix to a soft consistency with a little milk, then spread the mixture on top of the jam in the pastry case. Sprinkle the coconut over the mixture.

Put the flan tin on the preheated baking sheet, and bake the tart for 10 minutes. Reduce the temperature of the oven to 190°C/375°F/Gas 5, and bake for a further 20 minutes.

Fruit Salad

Fruit can be served raw in the hand or, as here, in a crunchy, juicy salad, and if you choose seasonally children should never be bored. You can add other fruit – kiwi, for instance – or leave some out.

Serves 4		Serves 96
1	orange	*12*
115g (4oz)	seedless grapes	*1.3kg (3lb)*
1 x 400g can	pineapple pieces	*1 x A10 (2.6kg) can*
115g (4oz)	glacé cherries	*675g (1½lb)*
225g (8oz)	eating apples	*2.7kg (6lb)*
225g (8oz)	bananas	*2.7kg (6lb)*
125g (4fl oz)	orange juice	*1.35 litres (48fl oz)*

Peel and segment the oranges over a dish. Cut into pieces and place in a large bowl (adding the juice that has collected in the dish as well). Halve the grapes and add to the orange. Add the pineapple pieces and their juice. Halve the glacé cherries, and add.

Peel the apples, if you wish, and core them and cut into bite-sized pieces. Add to the bowl. Stir, and leave to rest, covered, for about half an hour so that the flavours combine.

Just before serving, peel and chop the bananas into small pieces, and mix with the rest of the fruit and orange juice.

66 The dinners are good. I eat all of it and they make me feel full up. I like having healthy puddings and I'm called the banana man because I always have a banana instead of cake. 99

JAMES HERMAN, 8

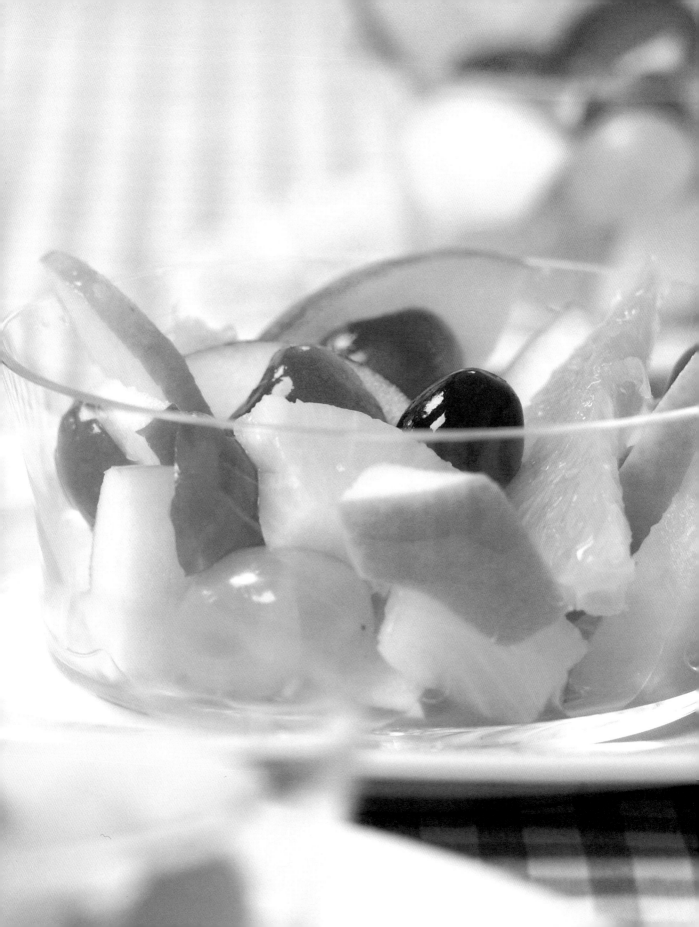

Apple Cobbler

This is one of my family's favourites. It is lovely and filling, especially when served with home-made custard (see page 245).

Serves 4		Serves 96
900g (2lb)	Bramley apples	*9kg (20lb)*
2	lemon slices	*24*
55g (2oz)	caster sugar	*450g (1lb)*
	Cobbler	
225g (8oz)	plain flour	*2.7kg (6lb)*
15g (½oz)	baking powder	*175g (6oz)*
55g (2oz)	butter or margarine	*675g (1½lb)*
55g (2oz)	caster sugar	*675g (1½lb)*
125ml (4fl oz)	milk	*1.4 litres (48fl oz)*

Preheat the oven to 180°C/350°F/Gas 4.

Peel, core and slice the apples. Cook over a low heat in a spot of water with the lemon slices until soft. Remove the lemon slices, put the apple into a deep tin, and stir in the sugar.

For the cobbler, sift the flour and baking powder into a bowl, then rub in the fat until the texture is like breadcrumbs. Add the sugar, and mix to a soft dough with the milk.

Turn the dough on to a floured table and roll out to 1cm (½in) thick. Cut out with a 6cm (2½in) cutter and arrange the rounds over the top of the fruit, overlapping. Brush with some extra milk.

Bake in the preheated oven for 30–35 minutes, or until golden brown.

> **❝** I want my children to learn the importance of good food at an early age, so I really appreciate that Mrs Orrey spends time talking to the children about what's good for them. They absolutely know that an apple is better than a bag of crisps. **❞**
> JO MANTLE, MUM

Manchester Tart

This will bring back memories to some of school dinners they had when they were children – and I mean in the nicest possible way!

Serves 4		Serves 96
	Pastry	
225g (8oz)	plain flour	*2.7kg (6lb)*
55g (2oz)	margarine	*675g (1¹/₂lb)*
55g (2oz)	vegetable shortening	*675g (1¹/₂lb)*
15g (¹/₂oz)	caster sugar	*175g (6oz)*
25ml (1fl oz)	water	*350ml (12fl oz)*
	Filling	
175g (6oz)	seedless raspberry jam	*1.8kg (4lb)*
700ml (1¹/₄ pints)	milk	*8.5 litres (15 pints)*
55g (2oz)	custard powder	*675g (1¹/₂lb)*
25g (1oz)	granulated sugar	*225g (8oz)*
25g (1oz)	good chocolate	*350g (12oz)*

Make the pastry as described on page 216, then roll out and use to line a 20–23cm (8–9in) loose-based flan tin. Chill for about 30 minutes. Preheat the oven to 200°C/400°F/Gas 6.

Neaten the edges of the pastry, line the pastry case with greaseproof paper and fill with baking beans (or dried beans). Bake blind in the preheated oven for about 15 minutes. Remove the beans and paper, and return to the oven to dry out for a further 5–10 minutes.

When cool, spread the base of the pastry case with jam.

To make a thick custard, put the milk in a saucepan, reserving some to mix with the custard powder and sugar into a runny paste. Gently bring the bulk of the milk to the boil, then pour it over the custard powder and sugar paste, whisking all the time. Return to the saucepan and gently cook for a further 2–3 minutes, stirring all the time. Cool the custard quickly by placing the saucepan in a bowl of cold water.

Pour the cooled custard into the jam-lined tart case. When the custard is cold, grate the chocolate and sprinkle it over.

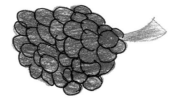

Bakewell Tart

A traditional Bakewell tart uses almonds, but because a lot of children have a nut allergy, I don't include it. The tart still tastes good, though!

Serves 4		Serves 96
	Pastry	
225g (8oz)	plain flour	*2.7kg (6lb)*
55g (2oz)	margarine	*675g (1¹/₂lb)*
55g (2oz)	vegetable shortening	*675g (1¹/₂lb)*
15g (¹/₂oz)	caster sugar	*175g (6oz)*
25ml (1fl oz)	water	*350ml (12fl oz)*
	Filling	
115g (4oz)	seedless raspberry jam	*1.8kg (4lb)*
	Sponge mixture	
115g (4oz)	butter or margarine	*1.1kg (2¹/₂lb)*
115g (4oz)	caster sugar	*1.1kg (2¹/₂lb)*
1	egg	*12*
115g (4oz)	plain flour	*1.1kg (2¹/₂lb)*
55g (2oz)	ground rice	*675g (1¹/₂lb)*
15g (¹/₂oz)	baking powder	*85g (3oz)*
125ml (4fl oz)	milk	*1.35 litres (48fl oz)*

Make the pastry as described on page 216, then roll out and use to line a 20–23cm (8–9in) loose-based flan tin. Chill for about 30 minutes. Preheat the oven to 200°C/400°F/Gas 6, and put a baking sheet in it to heat up.

Spread the pastry with the jam.

For the sponge mixture, cream the butter or margarine and sugar together, then beat in the egg. Sift the flour, ground rice and baking powder together and add to the creamed mixture. Beat well, adding sufficient milk to give a mixture that spreads easily. Spread the filling over the jam.

Bake in the preheated oven (on the hot baking sheet) for 10 minutes, then reduce the heat to 190°C/375°F/Gas 5. Continue baking for a further 20 minutes or until the filling is firm to the touch and golden brown.

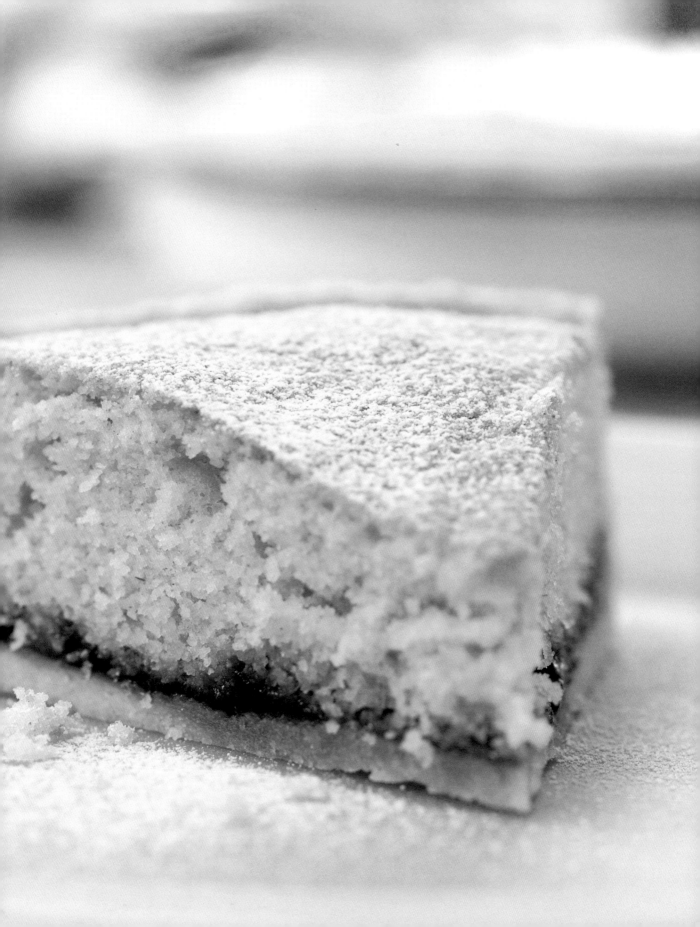

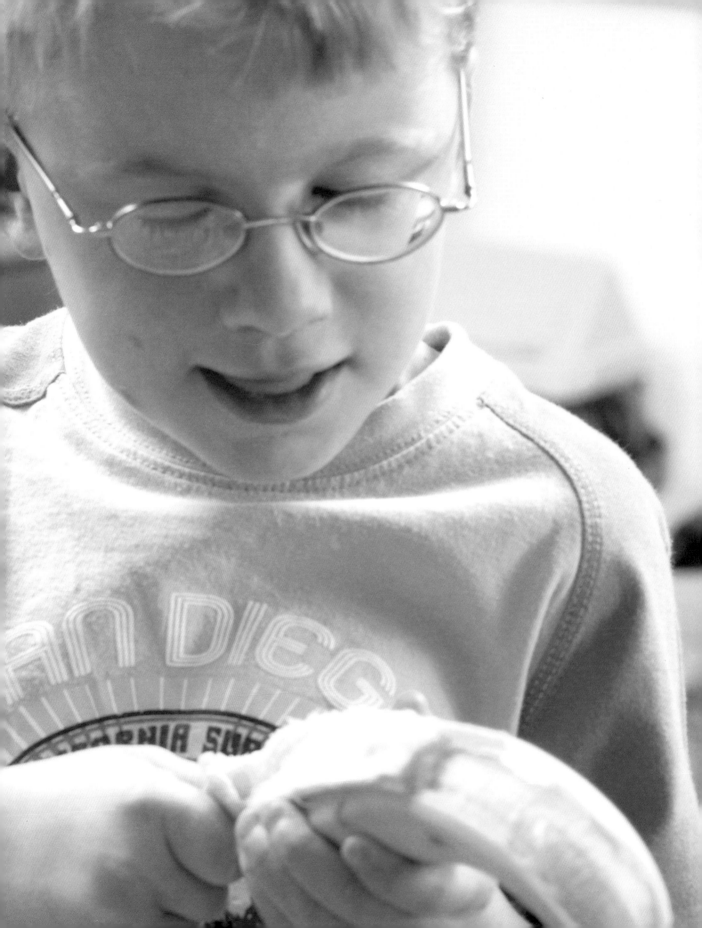

Apple and Banana Crisp

We use Bramley apples in all our apple puddings when they're in season. They're grown in Southwell, the home of the Bramley apple, about ten miles from St Peter's.

Serves 4		Serves 96
900g (2lb)	Bramley apples	*9kg (20lb)*
2	bananas	*12*
55g (2oz)	caster sugar	*225g (8oz)*
	Topping	
225g (8oz)	plain flour	*2.7kg (6lb)*
115g (4oz)	butter or margarine	*1.3kg (3lb)*
1/2 teaspoon	ground cinnamon	*2 tablespoons*
55g (2oz)	cornflakes	*675g (1 1/2lb)*
55g (2oz)	brown sugar	*500g (18oz)*

Preheat the oven to 180°C/350°F/Gas 4.

Peel, core and slice the apples. Peel the bananas and roughly chop. Cook the apples over a low heat with a spot of water until soft, then remove from the heat. Add the sugar and banana.

For the topping, sift the flour into a bowl. Cut the fat into cubes and rub into the flour along with the cinnamon until the texture resembles breadcrumbs. Slightly crush the cornflakes, and add them and the brown sugar to the flour. Mix again.

Place the fruit in a shallow baking tin – roughly 30 x 18cm (12 x 7in) – and top with the cornflake mixture. Bake in the preheated oven for 30 minutes.

Apple Crumble

According to Matthew Parker, this makes your tonsils tingle. For variety, you could use a mixture of plain and wholemeal flour for the crumble, and a mixture of caster and demerara sugar.

Serves 4		Serves 96
900g (2lb)	Bramley apples	*9kg (20lb)*
1	lemon or orange	*12*
55g (2oz)	caster sugar	*225g (8oz)*
	Crumble topping	
225g (8oz)	plain flour	*2.7kg (6lb)*
115g (4oz)	butter or margarine	*1.3kg (3lb)*
85g (3oz)	demerara sugar	*900g (2lb)*

Preheat the oven to 190°C/375°F/Gas 5.

Peel, core and slice the apples. Cut the rind of the lemon or orange into pieces. Put the apple and rind into a saucepan with a little water, and cook over a low heat until soft. Remove the rind. Add the sugar to sweeten, and put in an ovenproof dish.

For the crumble topping, sift the flour into a bowl. Cut the fat into cubes and rub into the flour until the texture resembles breadcrumbs, then mix in the sugar. Spread the crumble evenly over the fruit. Bake in the preheated oven for 35–40 minutes until lightly browned.

❝ My favourite is Yorkshire pudding and lamb with apple crumble and custard. ❞
RACHEL EDMONDS, 9

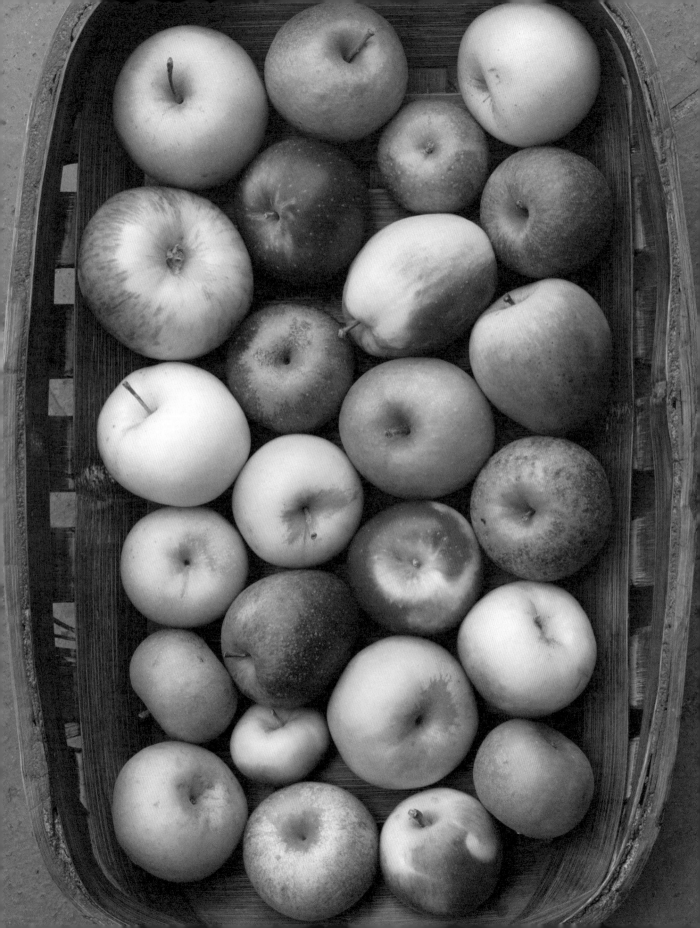

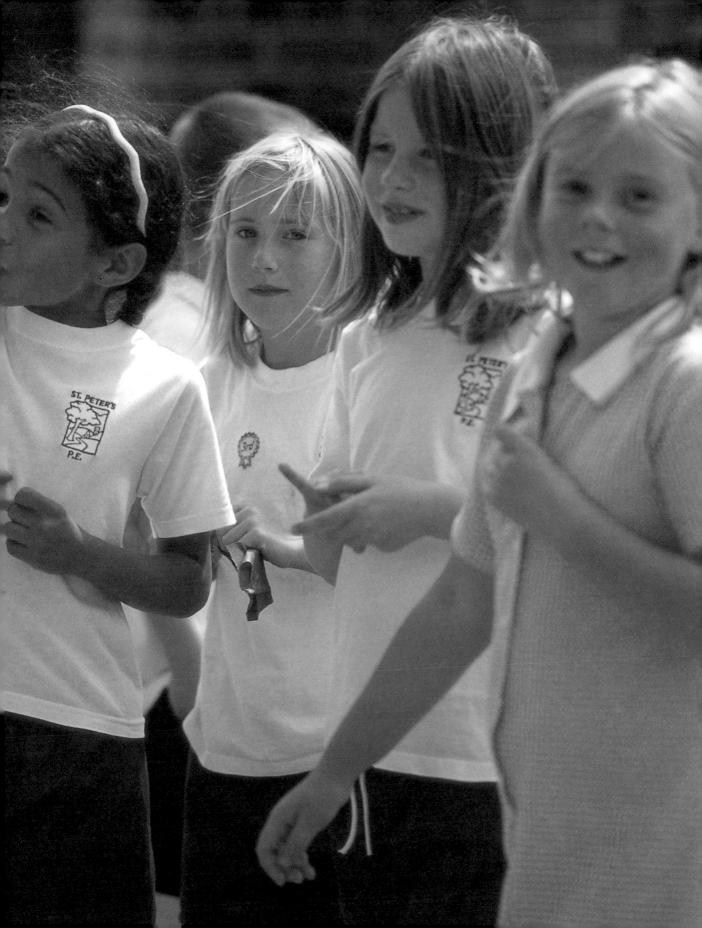

Oaty Apple and Sultana Crumble

A slight variation on the apple crumble, this recipe introduces a new texture to the children, by adding the oats.

Serves 4		Serves 96
900g (2lb)	Bramley apples	*9kg (20lb)*
55g (2oz)	caster sugar	*225g (8oz)*
	lemon juice	
225g (8oz)	sultanas	*1.3kg (3lb)*
	Crumble topping	
115g (4oz)	plain flour	*1.3kg (3lb)*
85g (3oz)	muscovado sugar	*675g (1½lb)*
115g (4oz)	rolled oats	*1.3kg (3lb)*
115g (4oz)	butter or margarine	*1.3kg (3lb)*

Preheat the oven to 180°C/350°F/Gas 4.

Peel, core and slice the apples. Add the sugar and a little lemon juice to stop them going brown, plus a small amount of water, and cook until soft. Transfer to a dish, something like a round 18cm (7in) dish. Sprinkle the sultanas over the apple.

For the topping, combine the flour, sugar and rolled oats in a mixing bowl. Melt the butter or margarine and add to the dry ingredients. Spread this mixture over the apples.

Bake in the preheated oven for 40 minutes until the topping is crisp.

66 The food is very, very nice, especially the puddings. If it gives the children a taste for proper food in the future, it must be a good thing. 99

SENIOR CITIZEN VISITING ON A WEDNESDAY

Jam Roly-Poly

This is a firm favourite in the winter term, served with fresh custard made with local milk.

Serves 4		Serves 96
350g (12oz)	self-raising flour	*4kg (9lb)*
1 teaspoon	baking powder	*55g (2oz)*
175g (6oz)	butter or margarine	*1.3kg (3lb)*
200ml (7fl oz)	milk	*2.4 litres (4¼ pints)*
350g (12oz)	raspberry jam	*4.2kg (9¼lb)*

If baking, rather than steaming, preheat the oven to 190°C/375°F/Gas 5.

Sift the flour and baking powder together, then coarsely grate the butter or margarine into the flour. (This can be done easily if the fat has been kept in the freezer.) Mix to a soft dough with the milk.

Roll the dough into a rectangle of about 30 x 20cm (12 x 8in). (Dinner ladies, divide the dough into 12 pieces first.) Lift on to a baking sheet covered with greaseproof paper. Spread the dough with jam, leaving a border of 1cm (½in) all round. Brush this border with water, and fold over a little dough at either end to seal the jam inside. Roll the dough up like a Swiss roll, using the greaseproof paper. Wrap in loose foil and seal with string at each end.

Bake in a roasting tray in the preheated oven for 1 hour. (Dinner ladies can steam roly-poly by placing in a deep and wide pan on a rack over boiling water, covering tightly and steaming for 1½ to 1¾ hours, topping up with water occasionally.)

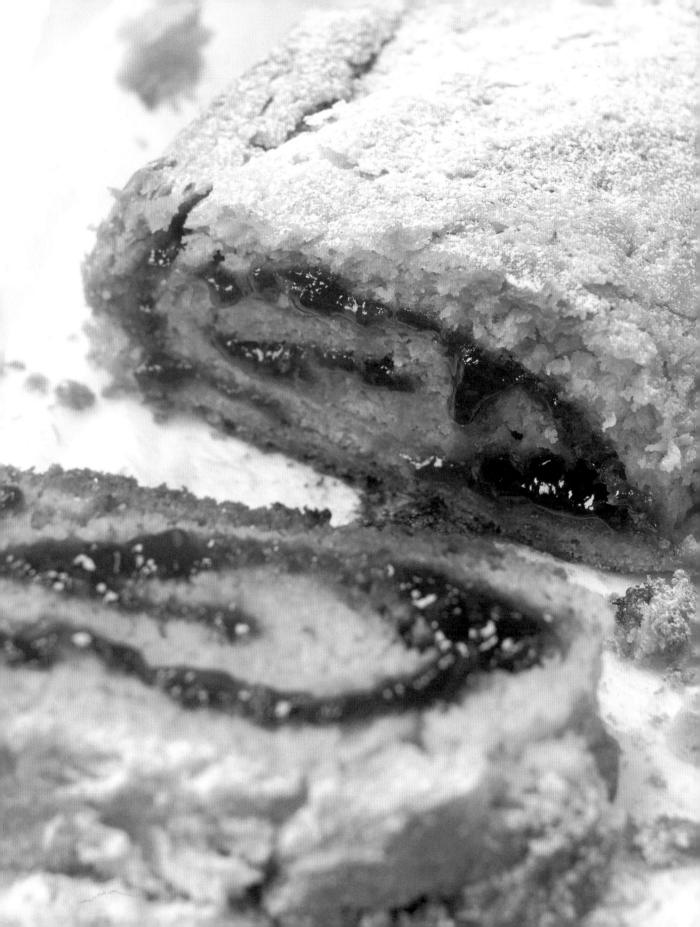

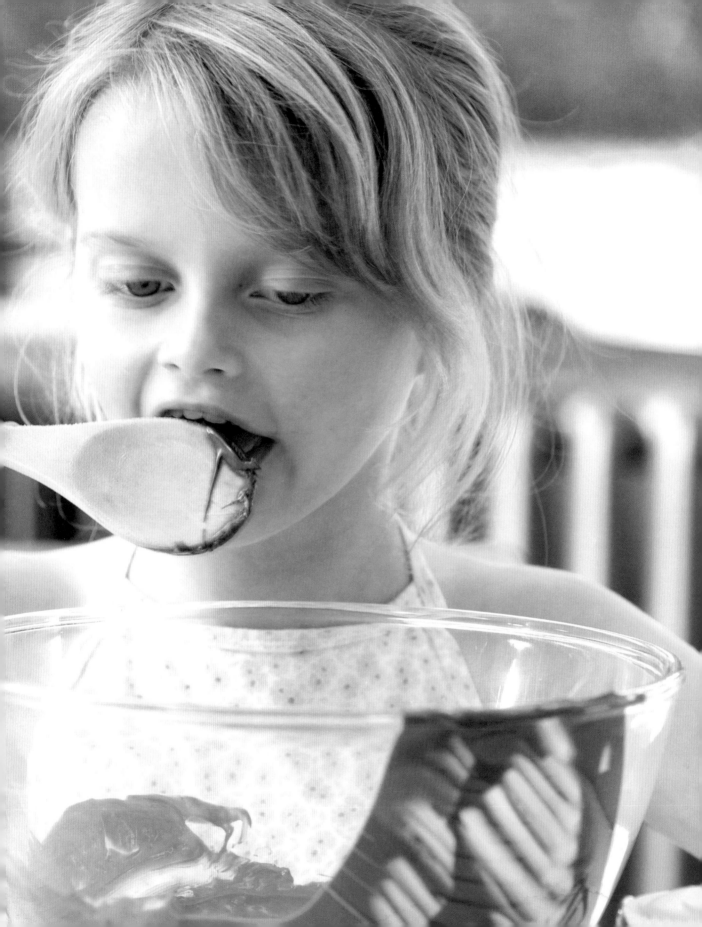

Gooey Chocolate Pudding

The children adore this, as do I, but the ladies in the kitchen don't like me when it's on the menu. It apparently makes a terrible mess with the washing-up water when they clean the tins and bowls! I tend to make this only in the winter.

Serves 4		Serves 96
	Sauce	
55g (2oz)	drinking chocolate	*425g (15oz)*
115g (4oz)	caster sugar	*1.3kg (3lb)*
600ml (1 pint)	water	*5 litres (9 pints)*
	Sponge	
2	eggs	*24*
50ml (2fl oz)	milk	*680ml (24fl oz)*
225g (8oz)	plain flour	*2.7kg (6lb)*
15g (½oz)	baking powder	*175g (6oz)*
15g (½oz)	drinking chocolate	*225g (8oz)*
115g (4oz)	butter or margarine	*1.3kg (3lb)*
115g (4oz)	caster sugar	*1.3kg (3lb)*

Preheat the oven to 180°C/350°F/Gas 4, and grease a deep 2.5-2.8 litre (4-5 pint) ovenproof dish.

Put the sauce ingredients into a large pan and boil briskly for about 5 minutes.

For the sponge, whisk the eggs and milk together in one bowl, and sift the dry ingredients together in another. Beat the butter or margarine and sugar together in yet another bowl. Gradually add the egg mixture to the fat and sugar mixture, a little at a time, alternately with the dry ingredients. Beat well for 1 minute. You may need to add a little more milk.

Put into the greased dish, and pour the hot sauce over the sponge mixture. Cover with a lid, and bake in the preheated oven for 35–40 minutes, or until when you insert a skewer it comes out clean. You might find it useful to place the dish on a baking sheet in the oven just in case of overflow.

Gooey Lemon or Orange Pudding

Make as for gooey chocolate pudding, except substitute the finely grated zest of 1 (12) lemon or orange in place of drinking chocolate in the sponge, and the lemon or orange juice in place of drinking chocolate in the sauce.

Bread and Butter Pudding

It has taken me a long time to reintroduce this to the children, but they now enjoy eating it. Perseverance does pay! There are ways in which you can liven up this basic pudding. You could add a few chopped dried apricots as well as sultanas to the bread, and you could infuse the milk first with a little lemon or orange zest. You could also sprinkle the top with a little demerara sugar.

Serves 4		Serves 96
25g (1oz)	butter	300g (10$\frac{1}{2}$oz)
175g (6oz)	bread, sliced	2kg (4$\frac{1}{2}$lb)
115g (4oz)	sultanas	1.1kg (2$\frac{1}{2}$lb)
40g (1$\frac{1}{2}$oz)	caster sugar	450g (1lb)
a pinch	grated nutmeg	5 teaspoons
3	eggs	36
600ml (1 pint)	milk	7.2 litres (12 pints)

Butter the bread frugally, keeping the crusts on. Cut each slice diagonally to form four triangles. Arrange the bread in layers in a well-greased deep tin, with the crusts to the bottom and the point of the triangle uppermost. Sprinkle the sultanas, sugar and nutmeg among the bread layers as you go.

Beat the eggs, and mix with the milk, then pour this custard mixture through a sieve over the bread. Allow to stand for 20–30 minutes for the custard to soak into the bread.

Meanwhile, preheat the oven to 180°C/350°F/Gas 4.

Bake the pudding in the preheated oven until the custard is set but wobbly and the top is beginning to brown and be crisp, about 25 minutes. Reduce the heat if the top browns too quickly.

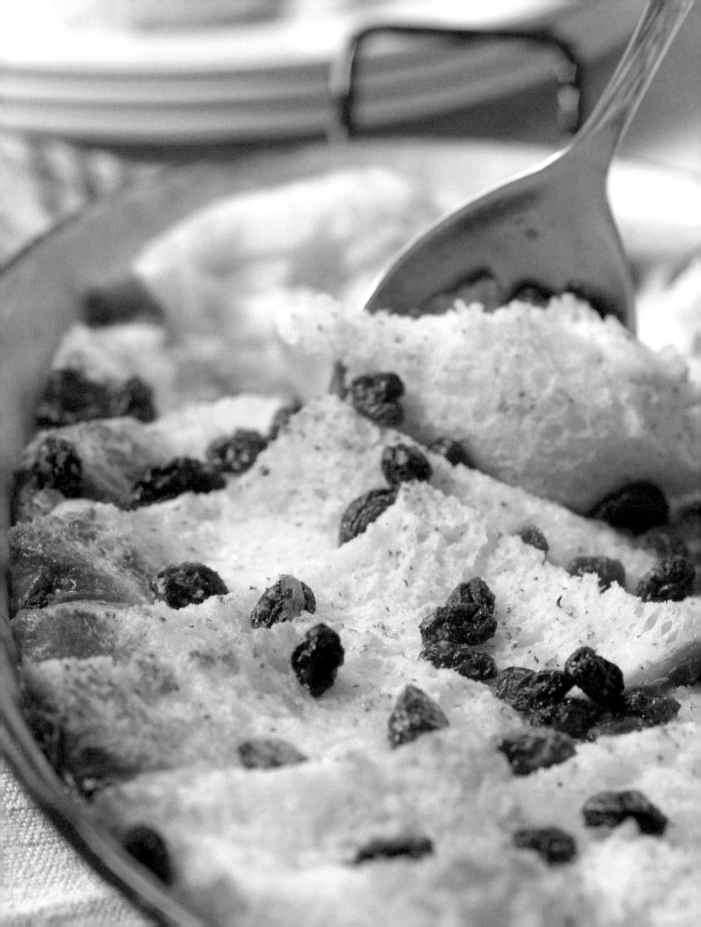

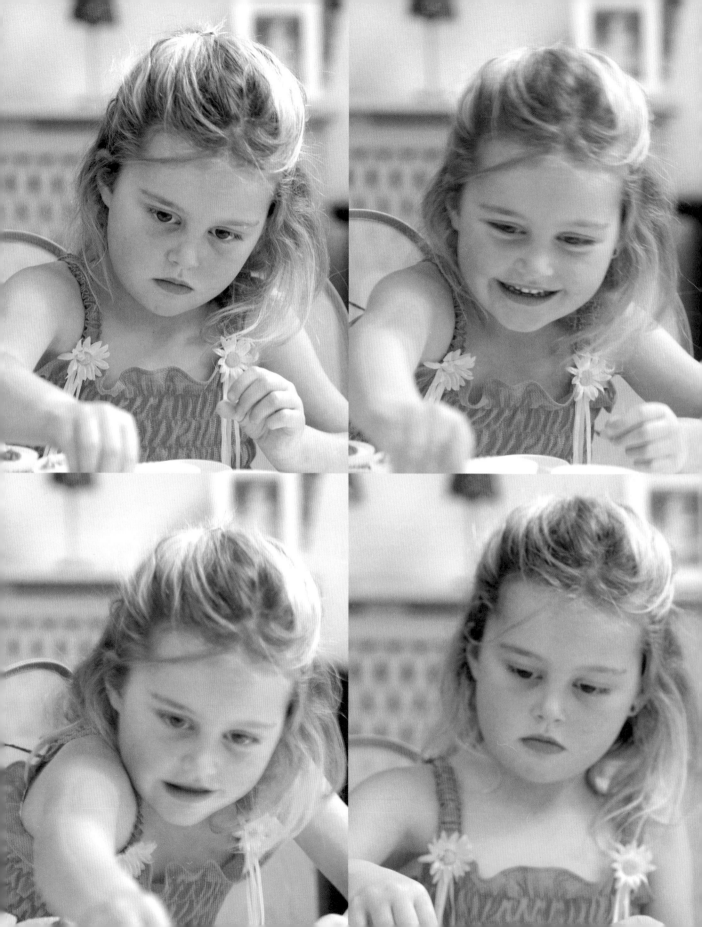

Jam Tart

The well-known British jam tart is everyone's favourite, I think, and is even better served with some home-made custard. By part-cooking the pastry case you get a crisp pastry bottom, not a soggy one. You can use lemon curd instead of jam.

Serves 4		Serves 96
	Pastry	
225g (8oz)	plain flour	*2.7kg (6lb)*
55g (2oz)	margarine	*675g (1½lb)*
55g (2oz)	vegetable shortening	*675g (1½lb)*
15g (½oz)	caster sugar	*175g (6oz)*
25ml (1fl oz)	water	*350ml (12fl oz)*
	Filling	
350g (12oz)	good jam	*4kg (9lb)*

Make the pastry as described on page 216, then roll out and use to line a 20–23cm (8–9in) loose-based flan tin. Chill for about 30 minutes. Preheat the oven to 200°C/400°F/Gas 6.

Neaten the edges of the pastry, line the pastry case with greaseproof paper, and fill with baking beans (or dried beans). Bake blind in the preheated oven for about 15 minutes. Remove the beans and paper, and return to the oven to dry out for a further 5–10 minutes.

Take out of the oven and spread jam into the pastry case. If you warm the jam in a saucepan first, you can just pour it into the pastry case.

Put back into the oven and cook for a further 20–25 minutes or until golden brown around the edges.

❝I think the dinners are lovely. It's like my mum's cooking.❞
ELIZABETH WRAGG, 10

Iced Apple Sponge

This is the favourite pudding of our deputy head, Mrs O'Leary. For a nice change, you could add some sultanas (about 25g/1oz) and a teaspoon of ground cinnamon to the basic cake mixture, and you could make the icing with lemon juice instead of water.

Serves 4		Serves 96
900g (2lb)	Bramley apples	9kg (20lb)
1	lemon	12
115g (4oz)	butter or margarine	1.3kg (3lb)
115g (4oz)	caster sugar	1.3kg (3lb)
2	eggs	24
225g (8oz)	plain flour	2.7kg (6lb)
15g (½oz)	baking powder	175g (6oz)
150ml (5fl oz)	milk	1.7 litres (3 pints)
140g (5oz)	icing sugar	1.8kg (4lb)
1 tablespoon	boiling water	175ml (6fl oz)

Preheat the oven to 180°C/350°F/Gas 4.

Peel, core and cut the apples into thin slices, then soak these in lemon juice.

Cream the butter or margarine and sugar together, then beat the eggs into this creamed mixture. Sift the flour and baking powder together into another bowl, and gradually add to the creamed mixture. Add sufficient milk to give a soft consistency, then pour the mixture into a greased shallow tin or a 22cm (8½in) springform cake tin. Place the sliced apples on the uncooked sponge, and bake in the preheated oven for 50–55 minutes. Remove and cool.

When the sponge has cooled, mix the icing sugar with enough boiling water to give a dropping consistency. Drizzle the icing over the top of the apple sponge, and serve with custard.

Rice Pudding

I used to have a job to get the children to eat this; now they cannot get enough. The reason, I believe, is the milk, which we get straight from the farm. Newfield Dairy, ten miles away from St Peter's, is a small family farm, and they have supported me right from the start. I regularly visit the farm to make sure everything is in order – and for a cup of tea.

Serves 4		Serves 96
115g (4oz)	pudding rice	*1.3kg (3lb)*
1.2 litres (2 pints)	milk	*14 litres (24 pints)*
25g (1oz)	butter	*225g (8oz)*
15g (½oz)	custard powder	*115g (4oz)*
25g (1oz)	caster sugar	*225g (8oz)*

Wash the rice in cold water. Drain and put in the top part of a double saucepan. Put boiling water into the bottom half of the pan, and sit the other pan on top. Add just enough cold water to cover the rice, cover and cook gently until the rice has absorbed the water. Add most of the milk and stir, then cover and leave over a gentle heat for about an hour.

Add the butter to the rice.

Put the custard powder, sugar and remaining milk in a bowl, and stir thoroughly. Add to the rice, mixing all the time, then cook for a further 10–15 minutes until thick and creamy.

❝I think school dinners are really tasty.❞
LYDIA MANTLE, 8

Toffee Tart

This is a favourite of grandparents, parents, teachers and children alike. They always want to take a slice home but I never have any left in the kitchen.

Serves 4		Serves 96
	Pastry	
225g (8oz)	plain flour	*2.7kg (6lb)*
55g (2oz)	margarine	*675g (1½lb)*
55g (2oz)	vegetable shortening	*675g (1½lb)*
15g (½oz)	caster sugar	*175g (6oz)*
25ml (1fl oz)	water	*350ml (12fl oz)*
	Filling	
100g (3½oz)	butter or margarine	*1.4kg (3lb 1oz)*
40g (1½oz)	plain flour	*675g (1½lb)*
250ml (9fl oz)	milk	*2.5 litres (4½ pints)*
55g (2oz)	caster sugar	*675g (1½lb)*
100g (3½oz)	golden syrup	*1.4kg (3lb 1oz)*
25g (1oz)	good chocolate	*350g (12oz)*

Make the pastry as described on page 216, then roll out and use to line a 20–23cm (8–9in) loose-based flan tin. Chill for about 30 minutes. Preheat the oven to 200°C/400°F/Gas 6.

Neaten the edges of the pastry, line the pastry case with greaseproof paper, and fill with baking beans (or dried beans). Bake blind in the preheated oven for about 15 minutes. Remove the beans and paper, and return to the oven to dry out for a further 5–10 minutes.

For the filling, melt the butter or margarine in a large pan, add the flour and cook, stirring, until sandy in texture and colour. Heat the milk in another small pan, and when hot, gradually whisk it in, along with the sugar. Cook, stirring all the time, until the mixture thickens then remove from the heat. Add the golden syrup and beat well.

Pour the mixture into the baked pastry case and set aside to cool. When the tart is cold, grate the chocolate and sprinkle it over.

Real custard

Give this a try, using organic eggs and milk. It's really creamy and lovely. You could use a vanilla pod instead of the vanilla essence.

Serves 4		Serves 96
4	egg yolks	48
25g (1oz)	caster sugar	350g (12oz)
15g (½oz)	cornflour	175g (6oz)
a few drops	pure vanilla essence	3 teaspoons
600ml (1 pint)	milk	7.2 litres (12 pints)

Beat the egg yolks and sugar together well in a large bowl. Mix the cornflour with just enough water to turn it into a paste (about 4 teaspoons for the home quantity), then stir it into the egg yolks along with the vanilla essence.

Bring the milk to the boil in a heavy-based saucepan. Gradually pour the hot milk into the egg yolks, whisking all the time. Return the mixture to the saucepan and heat gently over a very low heat, still whisking, until the custard thickens, about 5 minutes. (You could use a double saucepan, filling the bottom pan with hot water. Check the water level of the bottom pan periodically, and top up with boiling water if necessary.)

Serve straightaway.

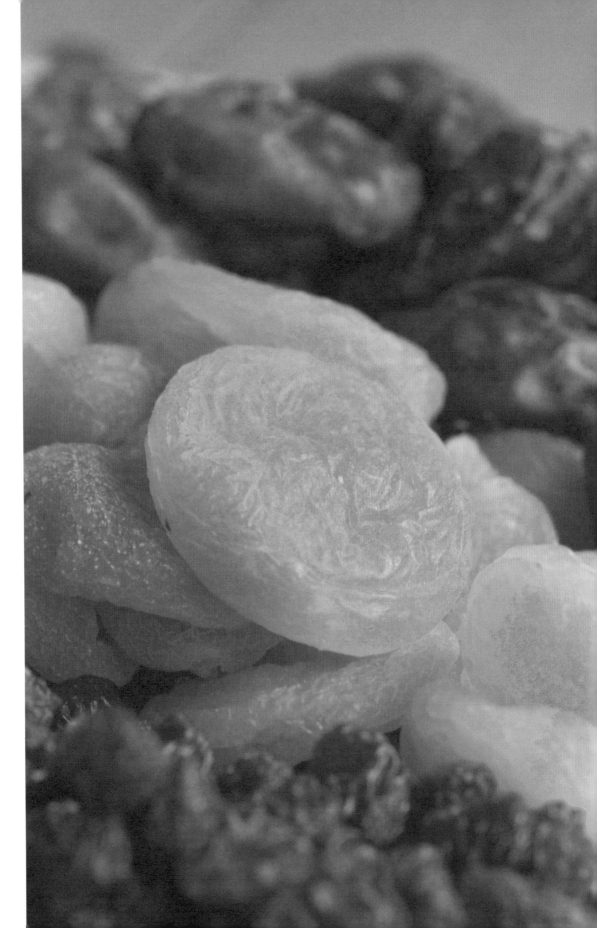

Cakes, Biscuits and Scones

Gingerbread

Ginger is an unusual taste for children, so this recipe is very mild. Use the gingerbread as a gentle introduction to this sweet spice.

Serves 4		Serves 96
225g (8oz)	self-raising flour	2.7kg (6lb)
2 teaspoons	ground ginger	8 tablespoons
2 teaspoons	mixed spice	8 tablespoons
115g (4oz)	dark muscovado sugar	1.3kg (3lb)
115g (4oz)	black treacle	1.3kg (3lb)
115g (4oz)	golden syrup	1.3kg (3lb)
115g (4oz)	butter or margarine	1.3kg (3lb)
2	eggs	24
150ml (5fl oz)	milk	1.8 litres (3 pints)

Preheat the oven to 160°C/325°F/Gas 3, and grease and line a 450g (1lb) loaf tin.

Sift the flour, ginger and mixed spice into a bowl. Melt the sugar, treacle, syrup and butter or margarine together for 5 minutes. Do not allow to boil.

Beat the eggs into the milk and add to the dry ingredients together with the melted mixture to make a soft batter.

Pour into the prepared tin and bake in the preheated oven for 35 minutes until springy to the touch. Cool in the tin.

Lemon Iced Sponge

This is another favourite of the children's, and one we cook in the summer. It has a refreshing lemony taste. You could make an orange iced sponge in the same way.

Serves 4		Serves 96
1	lemon	*12*
115g (4oz)	butter or margarine	*1.3kg (3lb)*
115g (4oz)	caster sugar	*1.3kg (3lb)*
2	eggs	*24*
225g (8oz)	plain flour	*2.7kg (6lb)*
15g (½oz)	baking powder	*175g (6oz)*
	milk	
	Icing	
1	lemon	*12*
225g (8oz)	icing sugar	*2.7kg (6lb)*

Preheat the oven to 180°C/350°F/Gas 4, and grease then line the base of a 20cm (8in) round cake tin.

Finely grate the lemon zest and squeeze the lemon juice into a small bowl. Cream the butter or margarine and sugar together in a bowl until smooth. Beat the eggs and then beat them into the creamed mixture. Sift the flour and baking powder, and add gradually to the creamed mixture, along with the finely grated lemon zest and the lemon juice. Add sufficient milk to give a soft dropping consistency.

Spoon into the prepared tin, and bake in the preheated oven for 30 minutes. Remove from the oven and leave to cool in the tin.

For the lemon icing, squeeze the juice from the lemon(s), and blend this with the icing sugar and enough water to form a good spreading consistency. Spread over the sponge when it has cooled.

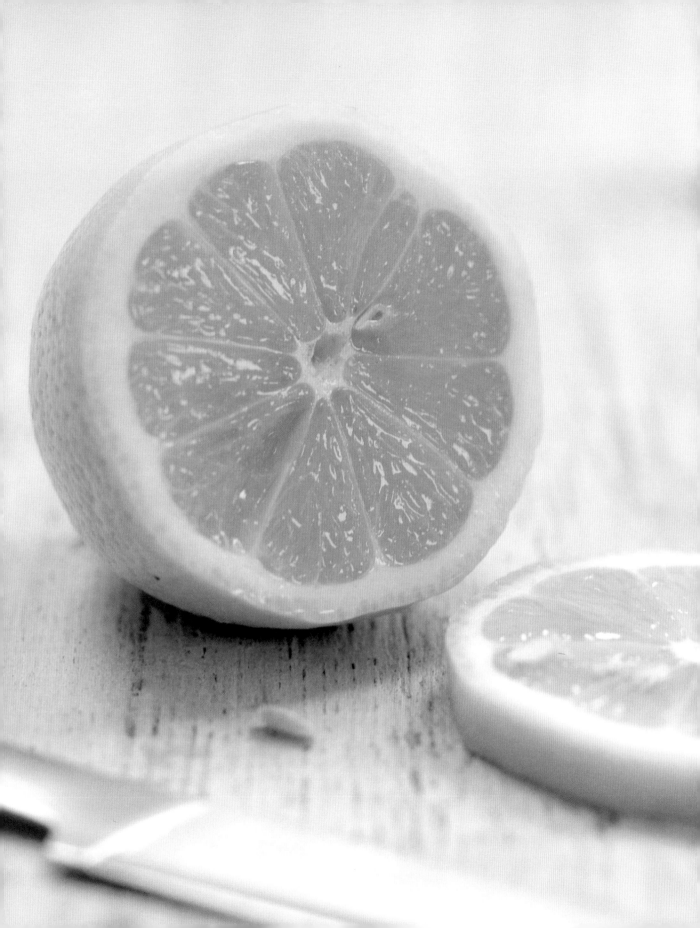

Muffins

We usually serve these with a glass of cold milk to excited gasps of, 'Ooh, it's muffins today!'

Serves 4		Serves 96
150g (5½oz)	plain flour	*1.8kg (4lb)*
½ tablespoon	baking powder	*6 tablespoons*
½ teaspoon	mixed spice	*6 teaspoons*
1	egg	*12*
125ml (4fl oz)	milk	*900ml (1½ pints)*
40g (1½oz)	caster sugar	*500g (18oz)*
55g (2oz)	butter or margarine	*675g (1½lb)*

Preheat the oven to 200°C/400°F/Gas 6.

Sift the flour, baking powder and mixed spice into a bowl, and set aside.

Whisk together the egg, milk and sugar in another bowl. Melt the butter or margarine and add to the milk mixture. Sift the flour mixture on top and briefly fold through – overlook the lumps, as these are what make the muffins rise. (You may need to add a little more milk for the larger quantity.) Add whichever combination of flavourings you choose, then spoon into muffin cases, filling them just to the top.

Bake in the preheated oven on a high shelf for 25–30 minutes.

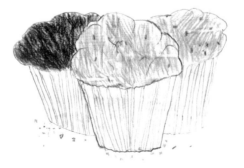

Banana

½ teaspoon	bicarbonate of soda	*6 level teaspoons*
175g (6oz)	bananas	*2kg (4½lb)*

Add the bicarb at the same time as the mixed spice. Mash the bananas and add along with the flour mixture.

Chocolate

25g (1oz)	drinking chocolate	*175g (6oz)*
½ teaspoon	vanilla essence	*6 teaspoons*

Add the drinking chocolate to the dry ingredients and the vanilla essence to the milk.

Chocolate Chip

55g (2oz)	chocolate chips	*450g (1lb)*

Add along with the flour mixture.

Apple

115g (4oz)	cooking apples	*900g (2lb)*

Peel, core and finely chop the apples. Add along with the flour mixture.

Cherry

55g (2oz)	glacé cherries	*450g (1lb)*

Wash the cherries, dry them thoroughly with a paper towel and chop them very small. Coat with a little flour, which will stop them sinking to the bottom of the muffins, and add along with the flour mixture.

Iced Fairy Cakes

The children could make these, and you could just supervise, popping the cakes into the oven when ready. When they are cooked, take them out and let the children decorate the tops.

Serves 4		Serves 96
115g (4oz)	self-raising flour	*1.3kg (3lb)*
115g (4oz)	butter or margarine	*1.3kg (3lb)*
115g (4oz)	caster sugar	*1.3kg (3lb)*
2	eggs	*24*
2¹/₂ tablespoons	milk	*450ml (16fl oz)*
1 teaspoon	vanilla essence	*50ml (2fl oz)*
	Icing	
115g (4oz)	icing sugar	*1.3kg (3lb)*
	boiling water	

Preheat the oven to 190°C/375°F/Gas 5.

Sift the flour into a bowl. Cream the butter or margarine and sugar together in another bowl, then beat in the eggs, alternately with the flour. Add sufficient milk to make a soft dropping consistency, and the vanilla essence.

Spoon the mixture into paper cases, filling each about two-thirds full. Bake in the preheated oven for 15–20 minutes.

For the icing, blend the icing sugar with a little boiling water, and mix well until smooth. Pipe or spread on top of the cakes.

Chocolate Fairy Cakes

Mix 55g (2oz) drinking chocolate (or 175g/6oz) with the flour. Add the same amount of drinking chocolate to the icing.

Lemon Fairy Cakes

Add the finely grated zest of 1 lemon and 1 tablespoon lemon juice to the sponge recipe (or zest of 12 lemons and 175ml/6fl oz lemon juice). Add the juice of ¹/₂ lemon (8 lemons) to the icing.

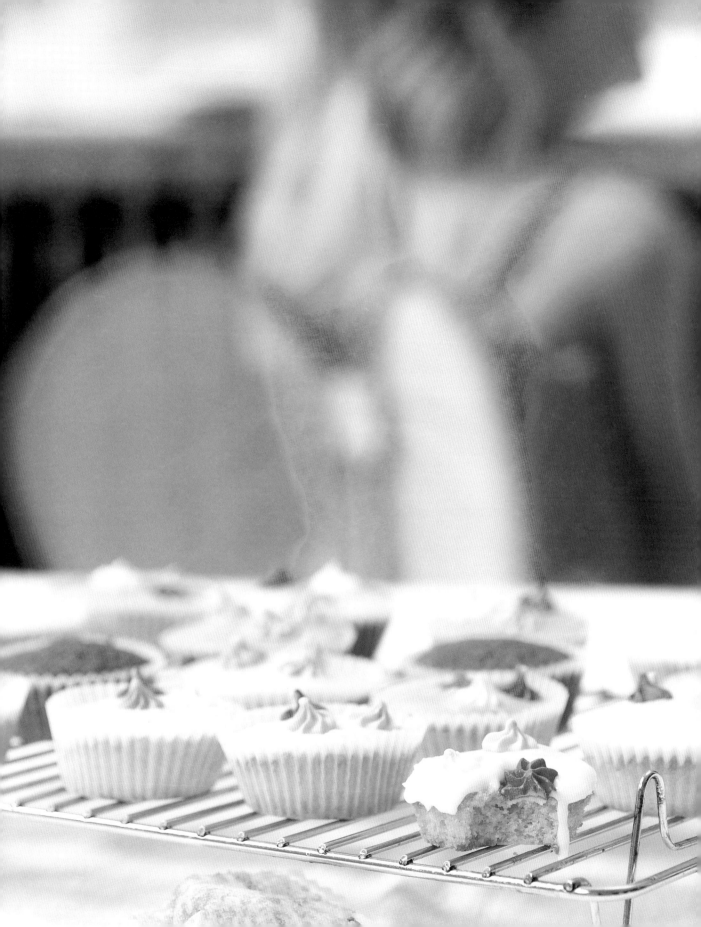

Chocolate Marble Sponge

The children always ask how I do this. It's actually very easy, but don't tell them, as they think I am quite clever!

Serves 4		Serves 96
115g (4oz)	butter or margarine	1.3kg (3lb)
115g (4oz)	caster sugar	1.3kg (3lb)
2	eggs	24
225g (8oz)	plain flour	2.7kg (6lb)
15g ($\frac{1}{2}$oz)	baking powder	175g (6oz)
85ml (3fl oz)	milk	1 litre (1$\frac{3}{4}$ pints)
55g (2oz)	drinking chocolate	175g (6oz)
2 tablespoons	warm water	6 tablespoons

Preheat the oven to 180°C/350°F/Gas 4, and grease a 20cm (8in) round cake tin.

Cream the butter or margarine and sugar together. Beat the eggs and beat them into the creamed mixture. Sift the flour and baking powder together. Add gradually to the creamed mixture, along with sufficient milk to give a soft consistency.

Divide the sponge between two bowls. Dissolve the drinking chocolate in the warm water, and stir this into one bowl of sponge mixture. Spoon the sponge mixtures alternately into the prepared tin, and blend the different colours with a skewer, but not too much – you want a marbled effect.

Bake in the preheated oven for 30–35 minutes or until springy to the touch.

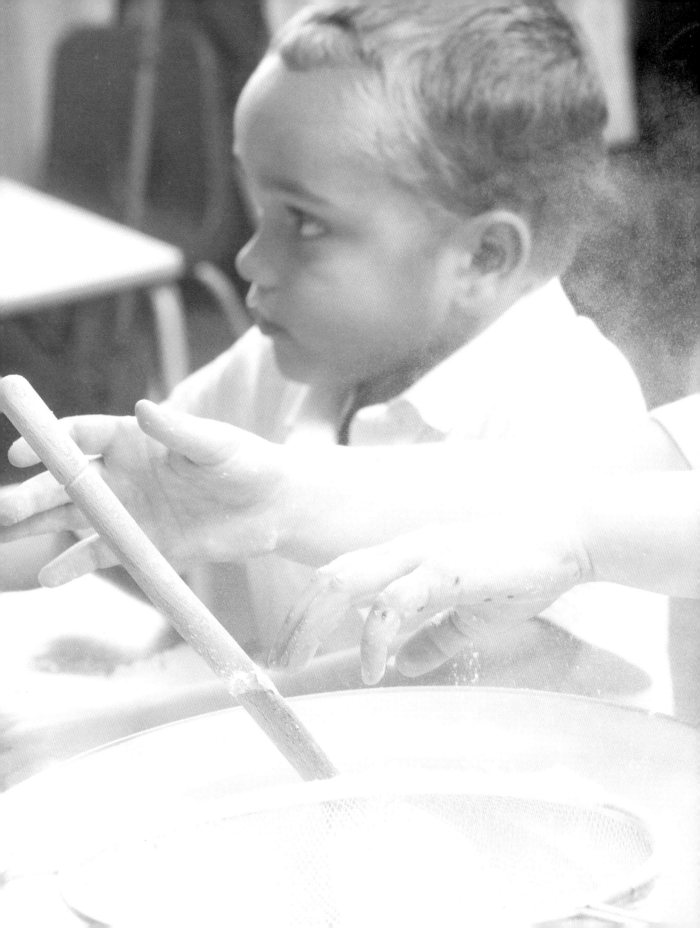

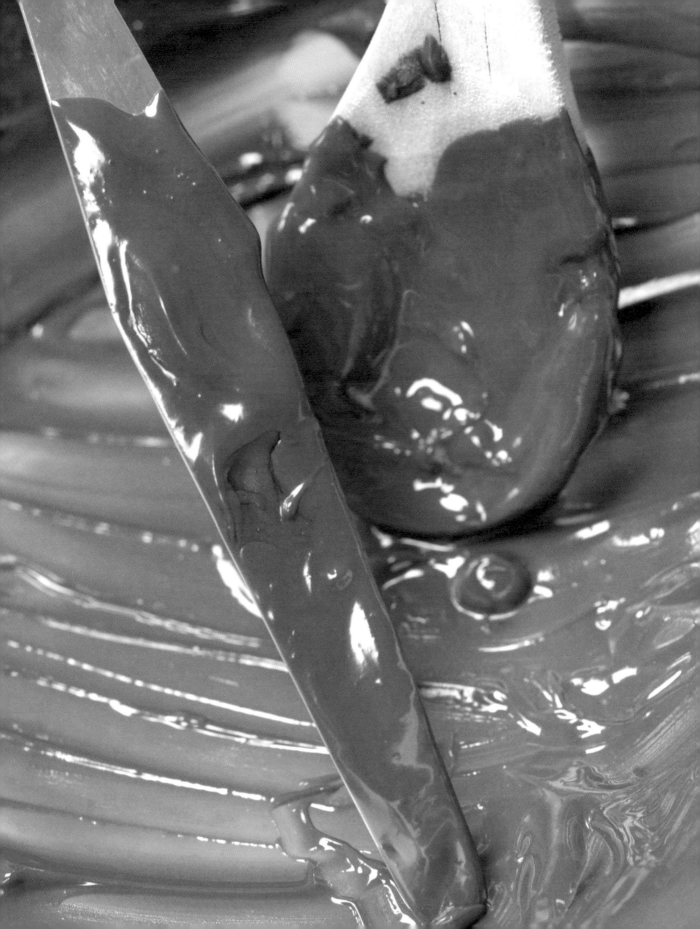

Chocolate Iced Sponge

I have reduced the sugar and it does not seem to have an effect on the recipe.
If you want it to be a little more luxurious, top with chocolate shavings.

Serves 4		Serves 96
115g (4oz)	butter or margarine	1.3kg (3lb)
115g (4oz)	caster sugar	1.3kg (3lb)
2	eggs	24
225g (8oz)	plain flour	2.7kg (6lb)
15g (¹/₂oz)	baking powder	175g (6oz)
85ml (3fl oz)	milk	1 litre (1³/₄ pints)
	Icing	
200g (7oz)	icing sugar	2.25kg (5lb)
55g (2oz)	drinking chocolate	225g (8oz)

Preheat the oven to 180°C/350°F/Gas 4, and grease a 20cm (8in) round or square tin.

Cream the butter or margarine and sugar together until smooth. Beat the eggs and beat them into the creamed mixture. Sift the flour and baking powder together, then add gradually to the creamed mixture, along with sufficient milk to give a soft dropping consistency.

Spoon the mixture into the prepared tin and bake in the preheated oven for 30 minutes. Remove from the oven, and leave to cool in the tin.

For the icing, blend the icing sugar and drinking chocolate with a little boiling water until a good spreading consistency. Spread on the sponge when cool, still in its tin.

Primary Choice Sponge

A real winner with the children, who chose the name. I don't put it on the menu all that often but, as I say to the children, a little of what you fancy does you good

Serves 4		Serves 96
	Sponge	
115g (4oz)	butter or margarine	*1.3kg (3lb)*
115g (4oz)	caster sugar	*1.3kg (3lb)*
2	eggs	*24*
225g (8oz)	plain flour	*2.7kg (6lb)*
15g (½oz)	baking powder	*175g (6oz)*
85ml (3fl oz)	milk	*1 litre (1¾ pints)*
	Topping	
85g (3oz)	butter or margarine	*900g (2lb)*
85g (3oz)	golden syrup	*900g (2lb)*
175g (6oz)	icing sugar	*1.8kg (4lb)*
1 tablespoon	drinking chocolate	*225g (8oz)*

Preheat the oven to 180°C/350°F/Gas 4.

To make the sponge, cream the butter or margarine and sugar together in a bowl. Beat the eggs, and then beat them into the creamed mixture. Sift the flour and baking powder together then add gradually to the creamed mixture. Add sufficient milk to give a soft consistency.

Put into a greased 20cm (8in) square cake tin and bake in the preheated oven until springy to the touch, about 30–35 minutes.

For the topping, melt the butter or margarine and the syrup together in a pan. Sift in the icing sugar and drinking chocolate, and beat until smooth. Spread on to the cake, and leave to set.

Carrot Cake

'Moist and sticky' is one child's description of this cake. I like it because it contains both vegetables and fruit.

Serves 4		Serves 96
140g (5oz)	butter or margarine	*1.6kg (3³/₄lb)*
140g (5oz)	soft brown sugar	*1.6kg (3³/₄lb)*
2 large	eggs	*24 large*
225g (8oz)	self-raising flour	*2.7kg (6lb)*
2 teaspoons	baking powder	*125g (4¹/₂oz)*
1	orange	*12*
175g (6oz)	grated carrot	*2kg (4¹/₂lb)*
¹/₂ teaspoon	vanilla essence	*6 teaspoons*
55g (2oz)	sultanas	*675g (1¹/₂lb)*

Preheat the oven to 190°C/375°F/Gas 5, and lightly grease then line the base of an 18cm (7in) square tin.

Cream the butter or margarine and sugar together until light and fluffy. Beat in the eggs and then fold in the flour, baking powder, orange zest and juice, grated carrot (patted dry first with kitchen paper if it looks watery), vanilla and sultanas.

Spoon into the prepared tin, and bake in the preheated oven for 45–50 minutes until golden brown. Cool in the tin before turning out.

When cold, coat with an orange icing, if you like (see page 248 and substitute orange juice for the lemon juice).

Banana Loaf

This loaf is ideal for us at school because you just have to slice it to serve. Bananas are great for energy, as well, just what the children need after working hard all morning. You could also ice this (add a little vanilla essence to the icing), if you like.

Serves 4		Serves 96
2	ripe bananas	24
175g (6oz)	butter or margarine	1.3kg (3lb)
175g (6oz)	caster sugar	1.3kg (3lb)
3	eggs	24
225g (8oz)	self-raising flour	2.7kg (6lb)
½ teaspoon	baking powder	2 tablespoons
½ teaspoon	vanilla essence	2 tablespoons
½ teaspoon	ground cinnamon	2 tablespoons
1	banana for decoration (optional)	12

Preheat the oven to 180°C/350°F/Gas 4.

Peel the bananas then crush with a fork. Beat together the butter or margarine and sugar, then add the eggs alternately with the flour and baking powder. Fold in the crushed banana, vanilla essence and cinnamon.

Pour the mixture into a greased 450g (1lb) loaf tin, and top, if liked, with long thin slices of banana. Bake in the preheated oven for about 40 minutes. Cool slightly then turn on to a wire tray. When cool, slice.

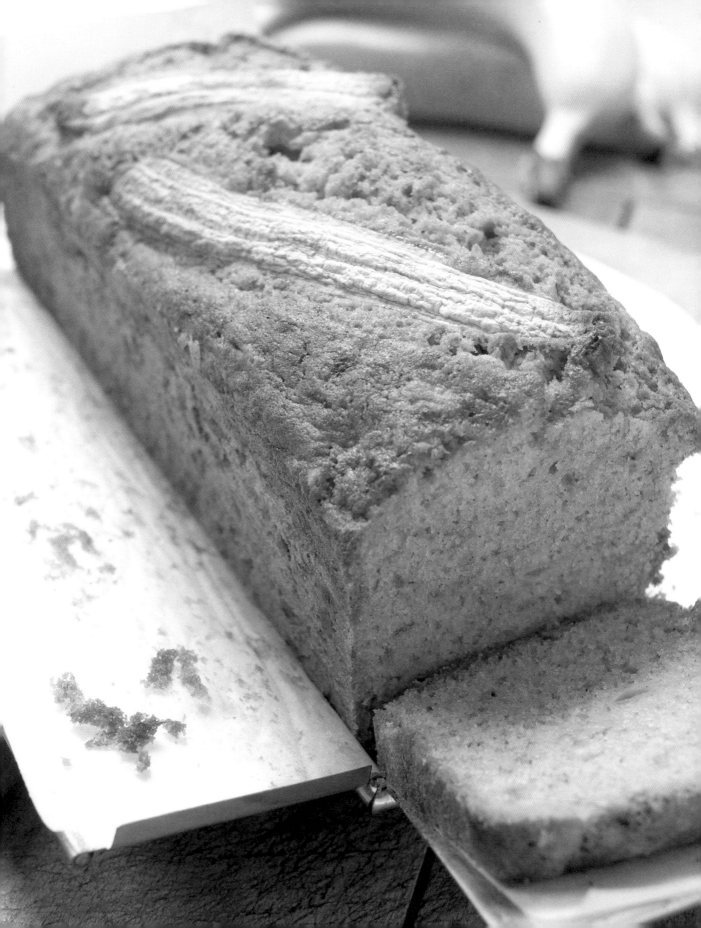

Mandarin Sponge

This is a twist on the conventional sponge recipe. You could decorate the top with freshly sliced orange as well as the mandarin segments.

Serves 4		Serves 96
1 x 312g can	mandarin segments	*1 x A10 (2.6kg) can*
115g (4oz)	butter or margarine	*1.3kg (3lb)*
115g (4oz)	caster sugar	*1.3kg (3lb)*
2	eggs	*24*
225g (8oz)	plain flour	*2.7kg (6lb)*
15g (½oz)	baking powder	*175g (6oz)*
	milk	
200g (7oz)	icing sugar	*2.25kg (5lb)*

Preheat the oven to 180°C/350°F/Gas 4, and grease then line the base of a 20cm (8in) cake tin.

Strain the mandarins, keeping both segments and juice.

Cream the butter or margarine and caster sugar together in a bowl until smooth. Beat the eggs and beat them into the creamed mixture. Sift the flour and baking powder, and add gradually to the creamed mixture, along with half the mandarin segments and sufficient milk to give a soft dropping consistency.

Spoon into the prepared tin, and bake in the preheated oven for 30–35 minutes, or until springy to the touch. Remove from the oven and leave to cool in the tin.

Gradually mix enough of the mandarin juice with the icing sugar to make it come together as an icing. Carefully stir in the reserved mandarin segments, pour over the cake and leave to cool and set.

Chocolate Slice

We serve this for a treat now and again. The slices are rather large, so you could cut them in half again to make 16 pieces.

Serves 4		Serves 96
175g (6oz)	plain flour	3.5kg (7lb 13oz)
125g (4½oz)	butter or margarine	2.7kg (6lb)
20g (¾oz)	caster sugar	225g (8oz)
	Topping	
25g (1oz)	butter or margarine	280g (10oz)
25g (1oz)	caster sugar	280g (10oz)
25ml (1fl oz)	milk	300ml (10fl oz)
115g (4oz)	icing sugar	1kg (2¼lb)
4 level teaspoons	drinking chocolate	175g (6oz)

Preheat the oven to 160°C/325°F/Gas 3, and grease a 20cm (8in) square tin.

Sift the flour into a mixing bowl and rub in the butter or margarine. Add the sugar and continue to mix until the ingredients come together as a stiff dough.

Roll out the mixture to fit the tin. Tip: this base can be hard to handle, so if you have a small rolling pin, finish rolling the base out once it's in the tin, or use the back of your hand to press to fit. Try to get it even. Bake in the preheated oven for 15–20 minutes, then leave to cool. Make sure you only lightly brown the base.

For the topping, place the butter or margarine, caster sugar and milk in a pan and melt over a low heat. Pour the melted ingredients over the icing sugar and chocolate in a bowl, and beat together for a minute. Spread the topping over the cooled base, and when cool and set, divide into portions.

Cornflake Crunchies

The children will love making these. Let them use their imagination and add things, such as raisins or chopped dried apricots or banana (remembering to chop them into small pieces).

Serves 4		Serves 96
55g (2oz)	butter or margarine	*675g (1½lb)*
115g (4oz)	milk chocolate	*1.3kg (3lb)*
125g (4½oz)	golden syrup	*1.3kg (3lb)*
25g (1oz)	caster sugar	*350g (12oz)*
115g (4oz)	cornflakes	*1.3kg (3lb)*

Melt the butter or margarine, chocolate and golden syrup together in a saucepan, then pour into a mixing bowl. Add the sugar, mix well, then add the cornflakes slowly.

Put into cake cases and pop into the fridge overnight.

When you go to the fridge the next morning you should have either eight or 96, unless you have two-legged mice, like I do . . .

"Dinners have always been nice at our school but now they are even better than before."
FRANCES JACKSON, 10

Chocolate Krispies

The children can help make these – if they don't eat the mixture before it gets into the paper cases.

Serves 4		Serves 96
55g (2oz)	butter or margarine	*675g (1½lb)*
115g (4oz)	golden syrup	*1.3kg (3lb)*
55g (2oz)	drinking chocolate	*175g (6oz)*
3 tablespoons	milk	*500ml (18fl oz)*
	vanilla essence	
115g (4oz)	Rice Krispies	*1.3kg (3lb)*

Melt the butter or margarine. Add the syrup, and boil for 1 minute. Take off the heat.

Sift the drinking chocolate into the syrup. Mix well, adding the milk, and vanilla essence to taste. Fold in the Rice Krispies, making sure they are all covered, then put into cake cases. Leave to cool and set.

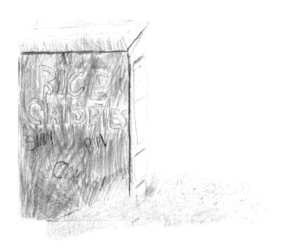

Chocolate Chip Cookies

Not something that immediately strikes you as 'healthy', but I am a firm believer in the occasional treat. The children fall on these when we make them, and I've also seen a few teachers in the rush ... For a different flavour, you could use chopped dessert chocolate instead of the bought chocolate drops.

Serves 4		Serves 96
225g (8oz)	plain flour	2.7kg (6lb)
15g (¹/₂oz)	baking powder	85g (3oz)
115g (4oz)	butter or margarine	1.3kg (3lb)
115g (4oz)	demerara sugar	1.3kg (3lb)
115g (4oz)	chocolate drops	1.3kg (3lb)
¹/₂ teaspoon	vanilla essence	25ml (1fl oz)
25ml (1fl oz)	milk	350ml (12fl oz)

Preheat the oven to 180°C/350°F/Gas 4.

Sift the flour and baking powder into a mixing bowl and rub in the butter or margarine until the mixture resembles breadcrumbs. Add the sugar, chocolate drops, vanilla essence and milk, and continue mixing until the ingredients come together as a soft dough.

Turn the mixture out on to a floured surface. (If cooking for 96, divide into 12 portions first.) Form into a roll approximately 10cm (4in) in diameter and slice into eight.

Place the cookies on parchment paper lined trays, and bake in the preheated oven for about 15 minutes until pale brown. Do not overcook.

You could of course make the cookies smaller, making about 12 instead of eight. Cook for a shorter time.

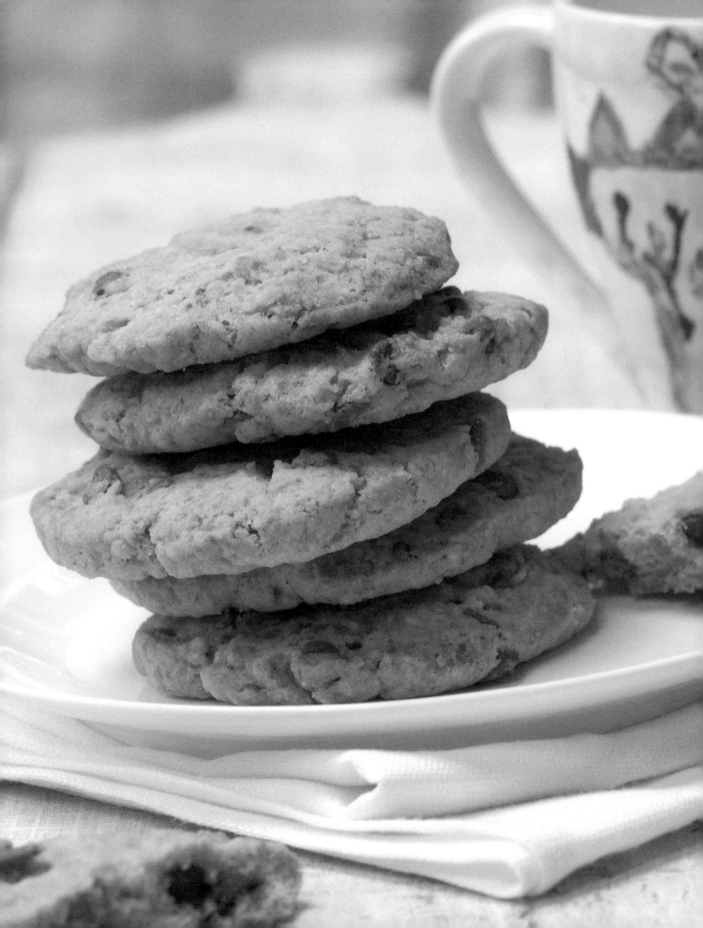

Oaty Chocolate Chip Cookies

Cookies are always a treat for kids, especially if they have helped you to make them. But I was surprised when parents who had come to help with the Christmas play last year asked, 'Have you made any of your cookies yet?' – at 9 in the morning!

Serves 4		Serves 96
175g (6oz)	plain flour	2kg (4½lb)
15g (½oz)	baking powder	115g (4oz)
55g (2oz)	rolled oats	675g (1½lb)
115g (4oz)	butter or margarine	1.3g (3lb)
115g (4oz)	granulated sugar	1.3g (3lb)
55g (2oz)	chocolate drops	650g (1lb 7oz)
25g (1oz)	golden syrup	350g (12oz)

Preheat the oven to 180°C/350°F/Gas 4.

Sift the flour and baking powder into a mixing bowl with the rolled oats, and rub in the butter or margarine until the mixture resembles crumbs. Add the sugar, chocolate drops and syrup, and continue mixing until the ingredients come together as a stiff dough.

Place the mixture lightly on a floured surface. Form into a roll approximately 9cm (3½in) in diameter and slice into eight. (Dinner ladies, divide up the mixture into manageable portions first.)

Place the cookies on to greaseproof paper on a tray, and bake in the preheated oven for 20–30 minutes until pale brown. Do not overcook.

Shortbread Biscuits

When I make these I use a 20cm (8in) square tin because to make it as individual biscuits would take me hours. I cut the shortbread while warm and cool it on a wire rack.

Serves 4		Serves 96
225g (8oz)	plain flour	2.7kg (6lb)
140g (5oz)	butter	1.7kg (3lb 15oz)
55g (2oz)	caster sugar	675g (1$\frac{1}{2}$lb)

Preheat the oven to 180°C/350°F/Gas 4, and grease the tin or baking sheet.

Sift the flour into a mixing bowl and rub in the butter until the texture is like breadcrumbs. Add the sugar and continue to mix until the ingredients come together as a soft dough.

Roll out to 1cm ($\frac{1}{2}$in) and cut out 8 or 96 biscuits using a 9cm (3$\frac{1}{2}$in) cutter. Or roll out into a square, put into a tin and neaten the edges.

Bake in the preheated oven for 10 minutes. Do not brown.

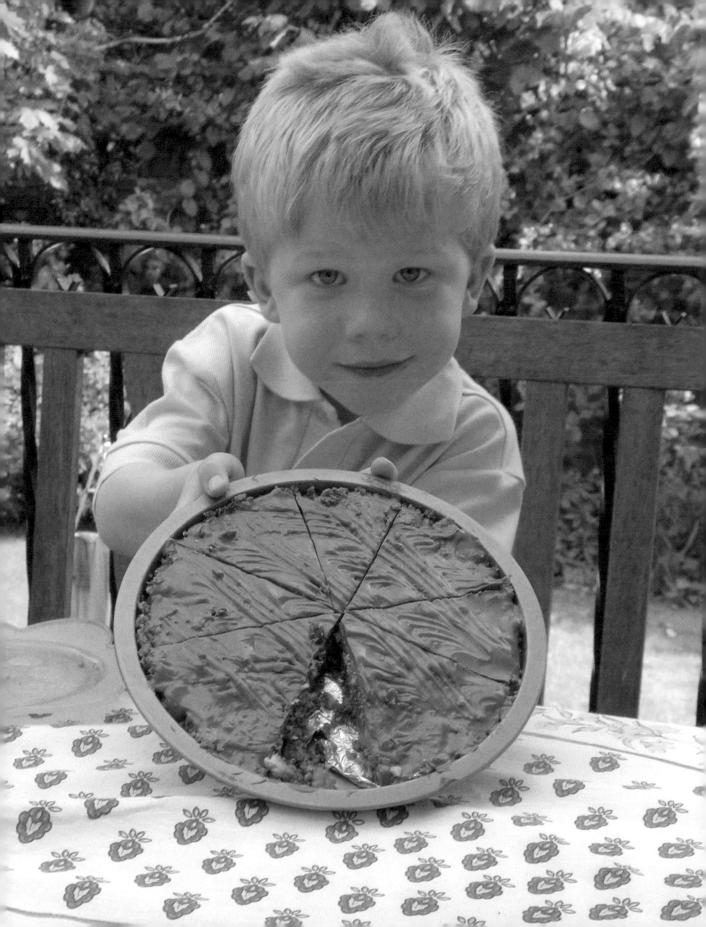

St Peter's Mud Pie

My dinner ladies love this one. They joke that it gives them an hour off because it doesn't need cooking. For that reason, it's also a dessert that's fun to make with kids.

Serves 4		Serves 96
225g (8oz)	digestive biscuits	*2.7kg (6lb)*
55g (2oz)	glacé cherries	*675g (1½lb)*
175g (6oz)	butter	*2kg (4½lb)*
1 tablespoon	drinking chocolate	*175g (6oz)*
115g (4oz)	caster sugar	*1.3kg (3lb)*
115g (4oz)	mixed dried fruit	*1.3kg (3lb)*
115g (4oz)	milk chocolate	*1.3kg (3lb)*

Break the biscuits into smallish pieces. Wash the glacé cherries of their sticky coating, dry them and chop into smallish pieces.

Melt the butter in a saucepan. Add the drinking chocolate and the sugar to the pan and mix together, then add the dried fruit, broken biscuits and chopped glacé cherries. Mix until all the ingredients are combined.

Line a 20–23cm (8–9in) round flan tin with foil, and pour in the mixture. Press down with the back of the spoon and place in the fridge for about 2 hours.

Break the chocolate into pieces and melt over an indirect heat (in a bowl set over a pan of simmering water). Pour the melted chocolate over the top of the chilled mixture, and spread, using a palette knife. Chill until set. Cut into pieces.

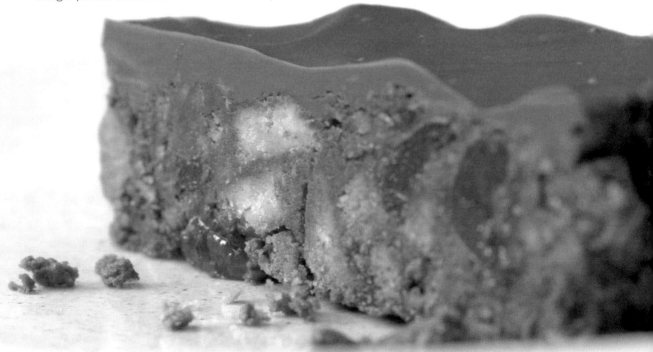

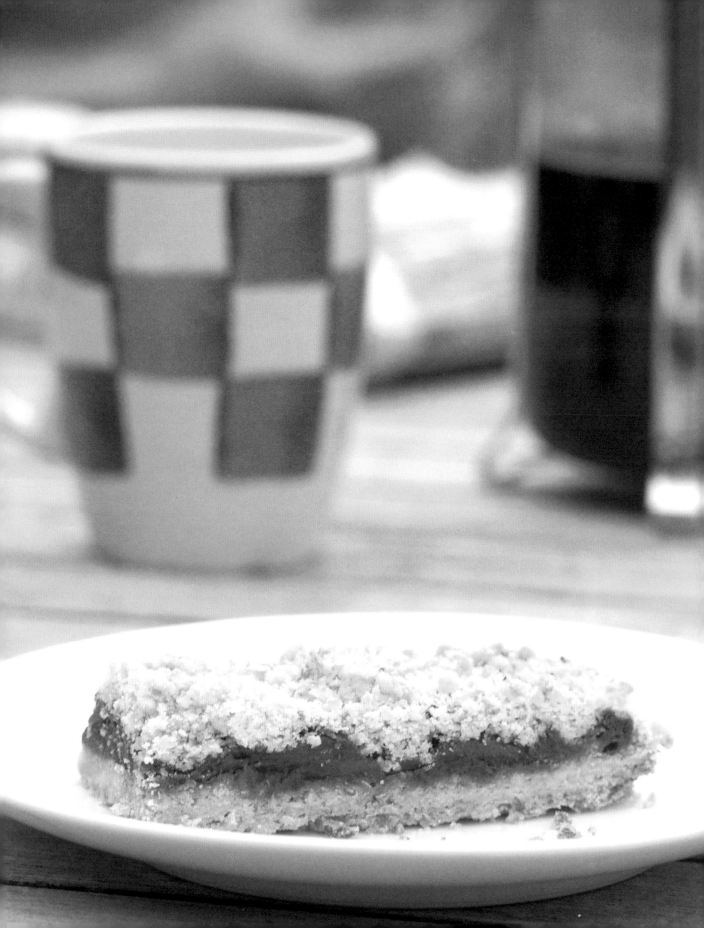

Dave's Date Slice

The head teacher David Maddison would have fired me if I hadn't put this recipe in the book. I'll let you into a secret: he can eat a whole one in a day! Instead of the dates, you could use dried apricots or figs.

Serves 4		Serves 96
350g (12oz)	pitted dates	4kg (9lb)
200ml (7fl oz)	water	2.5 litres (4½ pints)
1 large piece	lemon or orange rind	12 large pieces
140g (5oz)	butter or margarine	1.7kg (3¾lb)
225g (8oz)	wholemeal flour	2.7kg (6lb)
115g (4oz)	rolled oats	1.7kg (3lb)
85g (3oz)	dark brown sugar	900g (2lb)

Preheat the oven to 200°C/400°F/Gas 6. Grease a shallow rectangular cake tin, 28 x 18cm (11 x 7in).

Cook the dates in the water with the citrus peel until they are like jam (very soft), about 8–10 minutes. Discard the peel.

Rub the butter or margarine into the flour until the texture is like breadcrumbs. Add the rolled oats and sugar to make a crumble-type mixture.

Divide the crumble mixture in two and press half into the cake tin. Spread with the dates and cover with the remaining crumble.

Bake in the preheated oven for about 20–25 minutes, or until lightly browned. Cut into eight large slices or 16 small ones.

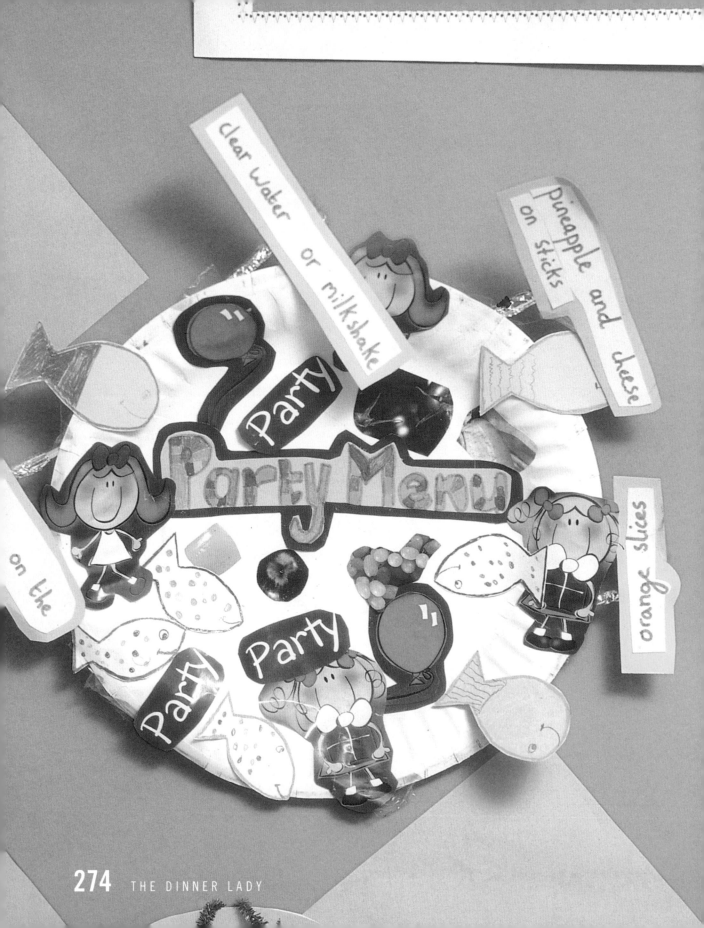

clear water or milkshake

Pineapple and cheese on sticks

Party

Party Menu

on the

orange slices

Party

Party

Flapjack

We sometimes serve this in the winter with a drink of warm milk. This quantity will fill one small shallow tin, about 25 x 20cm (10 x 8in) cut into eight, or five full-size flan tins cut into 20. You could add a few sultanas to the mixture, if you liked.

Serves 4		Serves 96
115g (4oz)	butter or margarine	*1.3kg (3lb)*
115g (4oz)	caster sugar	*1.3kg (3lb)*
85g (3oz)	golden syrup	*675g (1¹/₂lb)*
225g (8oz)	rolled oats	*2.7kg (6lb)*
1 teaspoon	vanilla essence	*10 teaspoons*

Preheat the oven to 180°C/350°F/Gas 4, and line the tin with baking paper.

Melt the butter or margarine, sugar and syrup together. Stir in the oats and vanilla essence. Spread the mixture into the prepared tin and bake for 25 minutes. Do not overcook.

Cut into portions and lift from the tin while still warm.

Cherry Shortcake

For a change, you could use sultanas instead of the cherries.

Serves 4		Serves 96
85g (3oz)	glacé cherries	*675g (1¹/₂lb)*
225g (8oz)	self-raising flour	*2.7kg (6lb)*
150g (5¹/₂oz)	butter	*1.8kg (4lb)*
70g (2¹/₂oz)	caster sugar	*850g (1lb 14oz)*
1 small	egg	*4 small*

Preheat the oven to 180°C/350°F/Gas 4, and grease then line the base of a 23cm (9in) loose-based flan tin.

Wash and dry the glacé cherries (this helps stop them sinking), then chop into small pieces. Sift the flour and baking powder together into a bowl. Rub the butter in until the mixture resembles breadcrumbs, then add the sugar and cherries. Whisk the egg and add this to the mixture. Mix together until it forms a smooth, thick paste.

Spoon the mixture into the prepared tin. Smooth the top, then bake in the preheated oven for about 25–30 minutes. Cut while still warm.

Scones

We make these in the summer when the children don't want or need a heavy pudding. You can make a variety of scones with this basic mix, adding sultanas or cherries, and even serving them with jam and cream. Note that the scone mixture should be soft. Avoid making too much at a time when oven space is limited, as the rising will take place in the warm kitchen instead of the oven.

Serves 4		Serves 96
225g (8oz)	self-raising flour	2.7kg (6lb)
1 teaspoon	baking powder	55g (2oz)
55g (2oz)	butter or margarine	650g (1lb 7oz)
55g (2oz)	caster sugar	650g (1lb 7oz)
150ml (5fl oz)	milk	1.7 litres (3 pints)

Preheat the oven to 220°C/425°F/Gas 7.

Sift the flour and baking powder into a bowl, then rub in the butter or margarine until the texture is like breadcrumbs. Add the sugar, and mix to a soft dough with the milk.

Turn the mixture on to a floured table and roll out to 2cm (³/₄in) thick. Cut into rounds with a 6cm (2¹/₂in) plain cutter (or, even nicer, cut into squares). Place on a greased baking sheet, and brush the tops with a little extra milk.

Bake in the preheated oven until well risen and lightly brown, about 10 minutes.

Sultana

Add 85g (3oz) sultanas for 4 portions, 900g (2lb) for 96 portions.

Sultana and Cherry

Add 55g (2oz) sultanas and 25g (1oz) chopped glacé cherries for 4 portions, 550g (1¹/₄lb) sultanas and 225g (8oz) glacé cherries for 96 portions.

Jam and Cream

Serve the plain scone with jam and cream. For 4 portions you will need 115g (4oz) jam and 175ml (6fl oz) whipped double cream. For 96 portions you will need 1kg (2¹/₄lb) jam and 2 litres (3¹/₂ pints) whipped double cream.

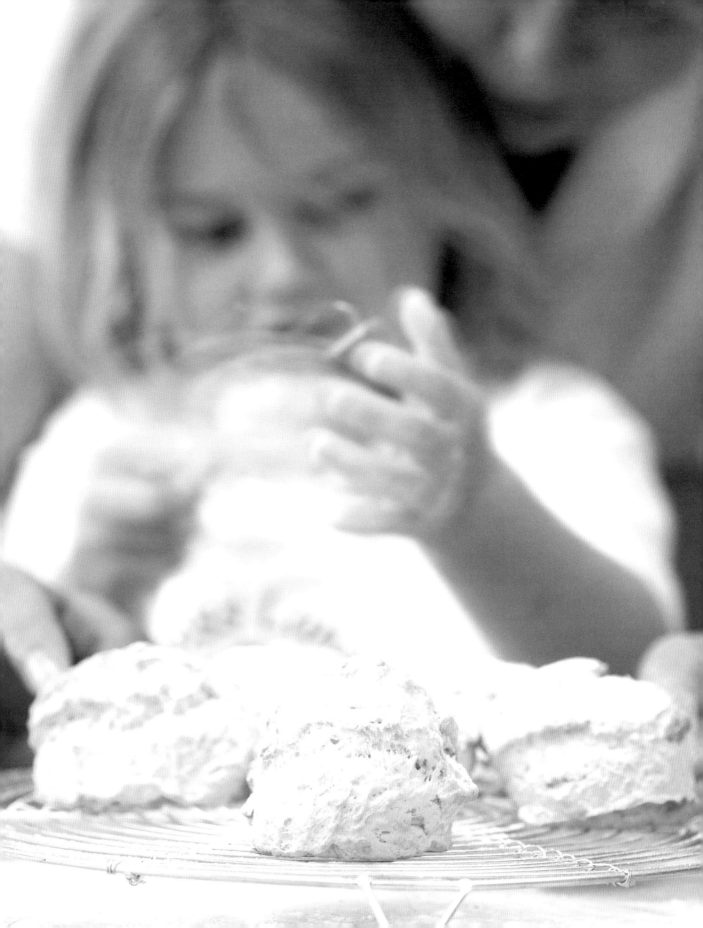

Access to Farms (ATF)
E-mail: janeth@rase.org.uk
www.farmsforteachers.org.uk

ALSPAC (Avon Longitudinal Study of Parents and Children)
Department of Community Based Medicine,
24 Tyndall Avenue,
Bristol BS8 1TQ
Tel: 0117 331 6731
E-mail: alspac-project@bris.ac.uk
www.alspac.bris.ac.uk

The British Dietetic Association
5th Floor,
Charles House,
148–9 Great Charles Street,
Queensway,
Birmingham B3 3HT

Caroline Walker Trust
PO Box 61,
St Austell PL26 6LY
Tel: 01726 844 107
www.cwt.org.uk

CASH (Consensus Action on Salt and Health)
Blood Pressure Unit,
St George's Hospital Medical School, Cranmer Terrace,
London SW17 0RE
E-mail: g.macgregor@sghms.ac.uk
www.actiononsalt.org.uk

Cooks in Schools
PO Box 47789,
London NW10 5ZU
Tel/fax: 020 8969 5723
E-mail: info@cooksinschools.org
www.cooksinschools.org

The Countryside Agency
Head Office,
John Dower House,
Crescent Place,
Cheltenham GL50 3RA
Tel: 01242 533222
E-mail: info@countryside.gov.uk
www.countryside.gov.uk

DEFRA (Department for Environment, Food and Rural Affairs)
Nobel House,
17 Smith Square,
London SW1P 3JR
Tel: 08459 33 55 77
E-mail: helpline@defra.gsi.gov.uk
www.direct.gov.uk

Focus on Food
Design Dimension,
Dean Clough,
Halifax HX3 5AX
Tel: 01422 383191

Food for Life
As for Soil Association opposite
www.foodforlifeuk.org
www.soilassociation.org/foodforlife

The Food Commission
94 White Lion Street,
London N1 9PF
Tel: 020 7837 2250
Fax: 020 7837 1141
E-mail: enquiries@foodcomm.org.uk

The Food Dudes
Professor Fergus Lowe,
School of Psychology,
University of Wales (Bangor), Brigantia Building,
Penrallt Road,
Bangor LL57 2AS
Tel: 01248 382210
Fax: 01248 382599

Friends of the Earth
26–28 Underwood Street,
London N1 7JQ
Tel: 020 7490 1555
Fax: 020 7490 0881
E-mail: info@foe.co.uk
www.foe.co.uk

The Health Education Trust
18 High Street, Broom,
Alcester,
Warwickshire
B50 4HJ
Fax: 01789 773915
www.healthedtrust.com

The Hyperactive Children's Support Group (HACSG)
71 Whyke Lane,
Chichester,
West Sussex PO19 7PD
www.hacsg.org.uk

International Association for the Study of Obesity (incorporating the International Obesity Task Force)
231 North Gower Street,
London NW1 2NS
Tel: 020 7691 1900
Fax: 020 7387 6033
E-mail: inquiries@iaso.org/obesity@iotf.org
www.iaso.org/www.iotf.org

Local Authorities' Caterers Association
Bourne House,
Horsell Park
Woking GU21 4LY
Tel: 01483 766777
E-mail: admin@laca.co.uk
www.laca.co.uk

Local Food Works
As for Soil Association opposite
Tel: 0117 914 2424
www.localfoodworks.org

Medical Research Council
20 Park Crescent,
London W1B 1AL
Tel: 020 7636 5422
Fax: 020 7436 6179
E-mail: corporate@
headoffice.mrc.
ac.uk
www.mrc.ac.uk

Milk for Schools
PO Box 412, Stafford,
Staffordshire ST17 9TF
Tel: 01905 642300
www.milkforschools.org.uk

Organic Networks
16 Ambrose Road,
Cliftonwood, Bristol BS8 4RJ
Tel: 0117 925 4929
E-mail: sbrenman@
organicnetworks.org

Organix Brands plc
Knapp Mill, Mill Road,
Christchurch BH23 8EW
Tel: 01202 479701
E-mail:
lizzie@organixbrands.com
www.babyorganix.co.uk

The Parents' Jury
94 White Lion Street,
London N1 9PF
Tel: 020 7837 2250
Fax: 020 7837 1141
E-mail: parentsjury@
foodcomm.org.uk

Pre-school Learning Alliance
The Campaign Team,
'Feeding Young
Imaginations',
69 Kings Cross Road,
London WC1X 9LL
Tel: 020 7833 0991
Fax: 020 7837 4942
E-mail: changinglives@
pre-school.org.uk
www.pre-school.org.uk/food

Soil Association
Bristol House,
40–56 Victoria Street,
Bristol BS1 6BY
Tel: 0117 929 0661
E-mail:
info@soilassociation.org
www.soilassociation.org

Sustain
94 White Lion Street,
London N1 9PF
Tel: 020 7837 1228
E-mail:
sustain@sustainweb.org
www.sustainweb.org

Unison
1 Mabledon Place,
London WC1H 9AJ
Tel: 020 7388 2366
www.unison.org.uk

Wellcome Trust
215 Euston Road,
London NW1 2BE
Tel: 020 7611 8888
E-mail:
contact@wellcome.ac.uk
www.wellcome.ac.uk

Further Reading

Joanna Blythman, **The Food Our Children Eat**, 4th Estate, 2000
Joanna Blythman, **The Food We Eat**, Penguin Books, 1998
Dr Stephen Davies and Dr Alan Stewart, **Nutritional Medicine**, Pan Books, 1987
DfEE, **Healthy School Lunches**, DfEE Publications, 2000
Sophie Grigson and William Black, **Organic**, Headline, 2001
Miranda Hall, **Feeding Your Children**, Piatkus, 1984
Brian Halvorsen, **The Natural Dentist**, Century Arrow, 1986
Felicity Lawrence, **Not on the Label**, Penguin Books, 2004
Harold McGee, **On Food and Cooking**, Unwin, 1986
Justin Sacks, **The Money Trail**, New Economics Foundation and The Countryside Agency, 2002
Eric Schlosser, **Fast Food Nation**, Penguin Books, 2002
Soil Association, **Food for Life**, Soil Association, 2003
Soil Association, **Where to Buy Organic Food**, Soil Association, 1998
Maryon Stewart, **Healthy Parents, Healthy Baby**, Headline, 1995
Mary Whiting, **Dump the Junk!**, Moonscape, 2002

At St Peter's we do not freeze anything, as everything is freshly made daily, but at home, if you're short of time, something prepared earlier and frozen can come in very handy (so long as you remember to defrost it in time!).

Foods to Freeze

Meat Raw meat in small cuts.
Raw and cooked meat in small shapes (burgers, meatballs).
Casseroled meats. Make sure that the liquid covers the solids when in the container.

Fish Raw, whole or filleted, but only if you know it is very fresh.
Very few cooked fish dishes, such as fishcakes.

Vegetables Only those with a low water content (no tomatoes, cucumbers, lettuces, radishes or other salad vegetables). Blanch tougher green and other vegetables for a few minutes first (to help keep their colour, flavour and texture).
Vegetable stews and purées, but preferably not potato.
Vegetable burgers and similar.

Fruits Raw, only berries, which open-freeze well (apart from strawberries, with their high water content).
Fruit purées, stewed fruits and fruit sauces.

Herbs Wash, chop and pack in water in ice-cube trays.

Cakes, biscuits and breads Ice, if relevant, only after defrosting.

Stocks Handy for soups and sauces.

Pastries Raw rather than cooked.

Sauces Tomato and other vegetable sauces particularly. Avoid egg-based sauces such as custard or mayonnaise, which will separate.

Butter and margarine Handy for making a quick pastry, as they can be grated into the flour.

Freezer Tips

- The freezer temperature should be –20°C. If higher than this, the foods will not freeze quickly enough.
- Pack dry goods tightly, to expel as much air as possible, preferably in freezer wrap. Wrap well, because any meat or fish that comes into contact with freezing air will get freezer burn.
- Label very clearly (otherwise you won't remember what was in that odd-shaped package).
- Remember that liquids expand by 10 per cent when frozen, so never over-fill plastic freezer containers (or the tops will be forced off in the freezer!).
- Defrost food slowly in the fridge, making sure it does not come into contact with other food.
- Add toppings or last-minute ingredients only when the dish has defrosted, and is being reheated.
- Reheat defrosted food very thoroughly.
- Try not to keep anything in the freezer for longer than three months.

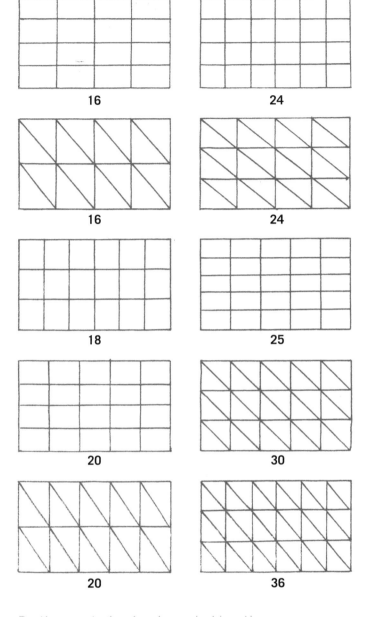

16 24

16 24

18 25

20 30

20 36

Portion control using large baking tins
Deep tin (7.5cm/3in deep) *Full tin*: 38 x 24cm (15 x 9½in)
Half tin: 24 x 18cm (9½ x 7in)
Shallow tin (2.5cm/1in deep) *Full tin*: 38 x 24cm (15 x 9½in)
Half tin: 24 x 18cm (9½ x 7in)

A Note about Recipe Proportions

The recipe proportions may sometimes look arbitrary, but the quantities for four and for 96 should not be compared. The quantities quoted work for four and, separately, for 96.

THERE ARE SO MANY PEOPLE I want to thank for their support, friendship and for just being there to listen to me while I rant on about food and what is happening in our schools.

Most of all I would like to thank my husband George Orrey for his love and total support and understanding of what I am trying to achieve and for the thirty years we have spent together.

My thanks to my Mum, Dad and Mum-in-law, who always have a special place in my heart.

To all the staff, governing body and the children of St Peter's Primary School.

And to another special person in my life – a man who gave me the chance to 'know what is possible' – St Peter's head teacher, David Maddison, who listened, encouraged and gave me a belief in myself I did not know I had. May our friendship last always.

I would also like to take this opportunity to say a big thank you to the following people:

To everyone at the Soil Association.

To my agent and friend Lizzy Kremer, to Susan Fleming, who has become a friend and without whose expertise this book would not have been written. Special thanks to Diana Beaumont for her faith in me, Fiona Andreanelli, Alison Barrow, Sally Gaminara, Patrick Janson-Smith, Liz Laczynska, Phil Lord, Katrina Whone, and everyone else at Transworld for making me feel at ease and for doing such a fantastic job. To Jamie for his friendship, to Robin Williams – sorry, Matthews – for the photographs, and to Caroline Marson, home economist, and Helen Crawley, nutritionist.

Many thanks go to Lizzie Vann, whom I first met at the Soil Association and continue to work with.

I am especially grateful to the ladies in my kitchen, Chris, Alison, Jane and Christine, without whose loyalty, friendship, never-ending enthusiasm and hard work we would not be where we are today.

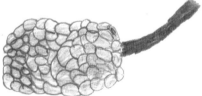

Lastly, this book is for all the dinner ladies I have met on my travels across the country.
I hope you enjoy this book.
WE WILL GET THERE!

Picture Acknowledgements

All photographs by Robin Matthews unless otherwise credited.

p.32 © Pepin Press; p.35: (top) © Hulton Archive/Getty, (bottom) © Time & Life Pictures/Getty; pp.48/9 Foodfolio/Alamy; p.59: © Hulton Archive/Getty; p.63 © Pepin Press; p.71: © O'Brien Productions/Corbis; p.82: © PhotoAlto/Getty; p.86: Fabio de Paola; p.107: © Terry W. Eggers/Corbis; p.109: © Food Pix/Getty; p.112: © Pepin Press; p.113: © Pepin Press; pp.116/17: © The Image Bank/Getty; p.122: © Stone/Getty; p.138: © www.britainonview.com/Adam Swai; p.166: © David Murray/Dorling Kindersley; p.175: © Pepin Press; p.191: © Pepin Press; p.231: © Botanica/Getty; p.270: Caroline Marson

Illustrations

Lauren Prideaux: pp.1, 30
Francesca Halter: p.25
Thomas Park: pp.26, 50, 221, 225, 259
Abby Ashmore: p.28
Elizabeth Whitworth: p.31
Jake Booth: p.38
Daniel Pereira: p.51
Charlotte Hepples: p.65
Adam Hartfield: p.73
Jessica Morrell: p.77
Tom Crossland: p.92
Adam Phillips: p.120
Jacob Morton: p.135
Danny Lord: pp.140, 250, 265
Rebecca Tupholme: p.150
Helena Bradbury: p.165
Dominic Wealthall: p.205, 287
Ben Cree: p.207
Rebecca Orrey: p.212